100 Essential Steps

for

Healthy Living

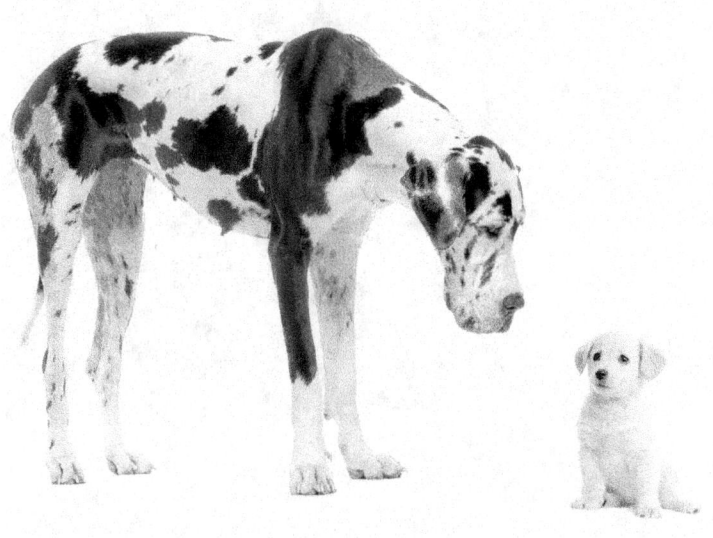

Try not to critically compare yourself to others

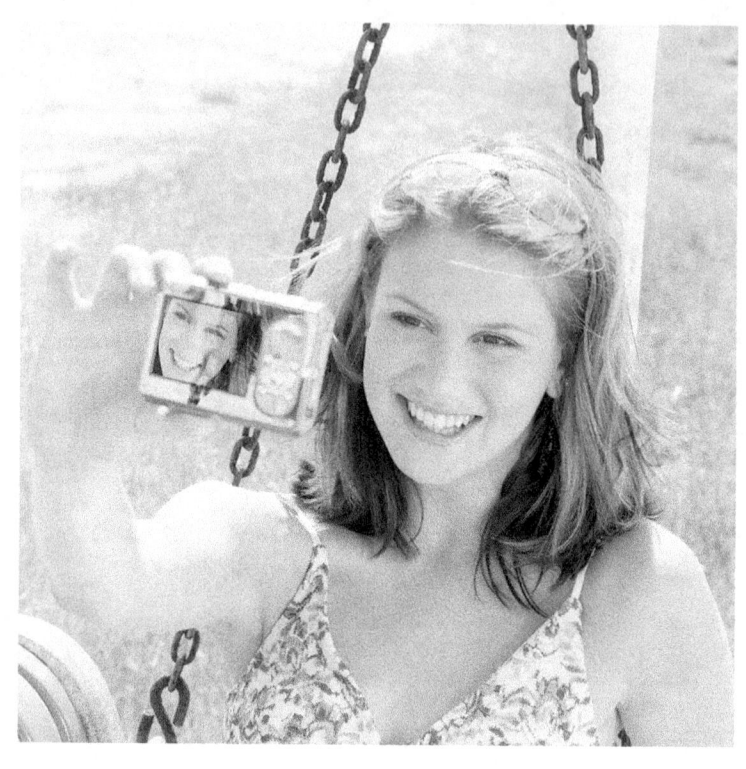

Happiness depends upon your own approval

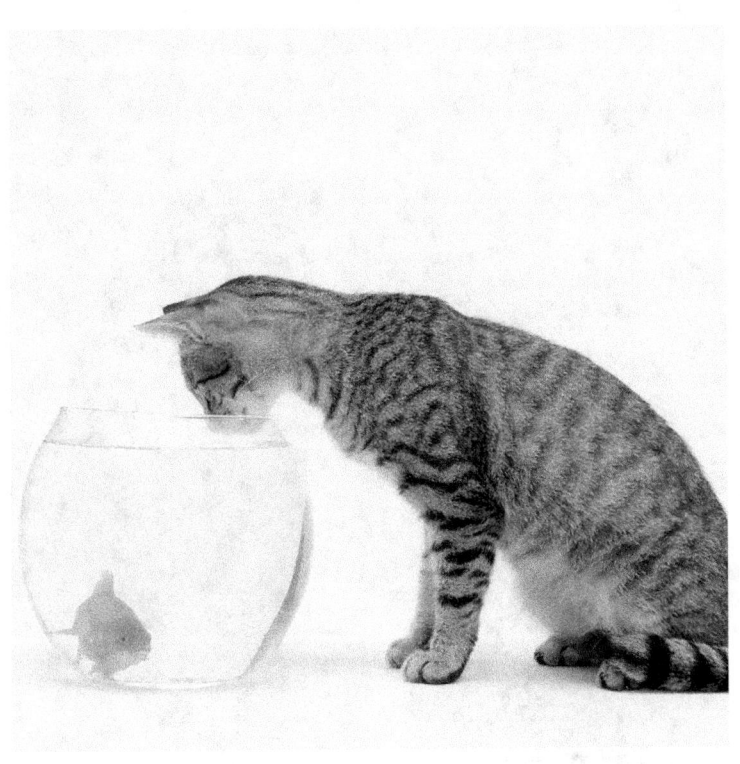

Try to include a healthy source of protein in every meal

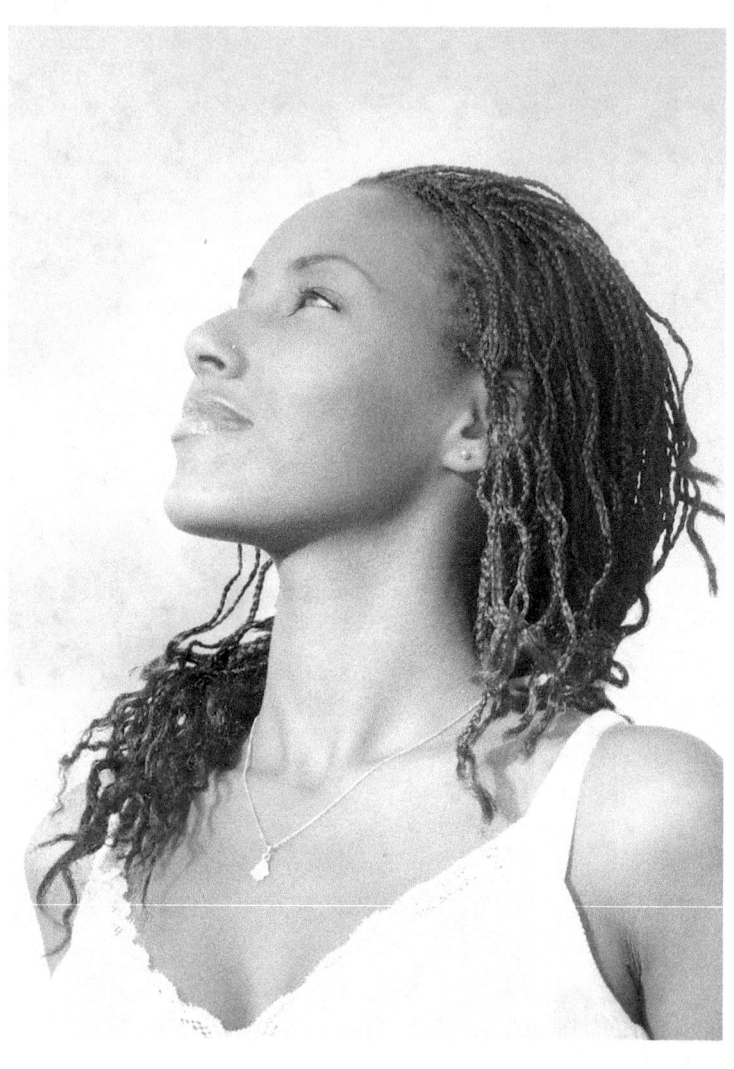

True beauty is revealed from the light within us

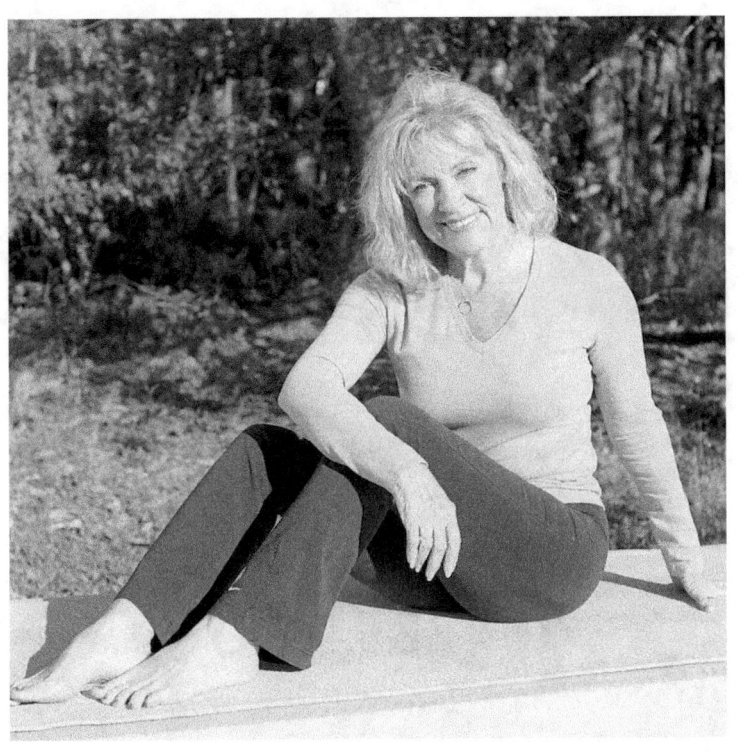

Measure your age by your health not by your years

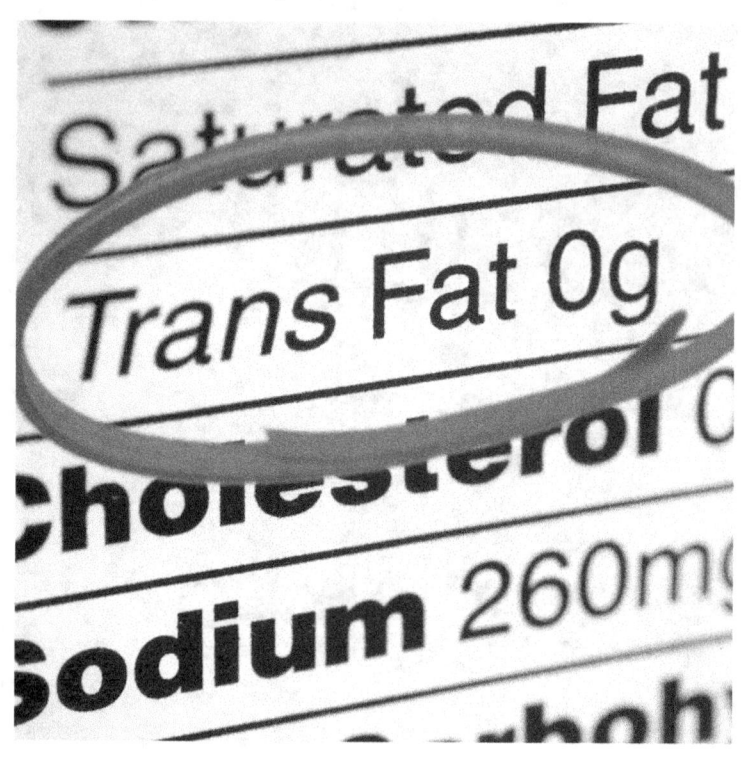

Educate yourself on the nutritional content
of the foods you eat

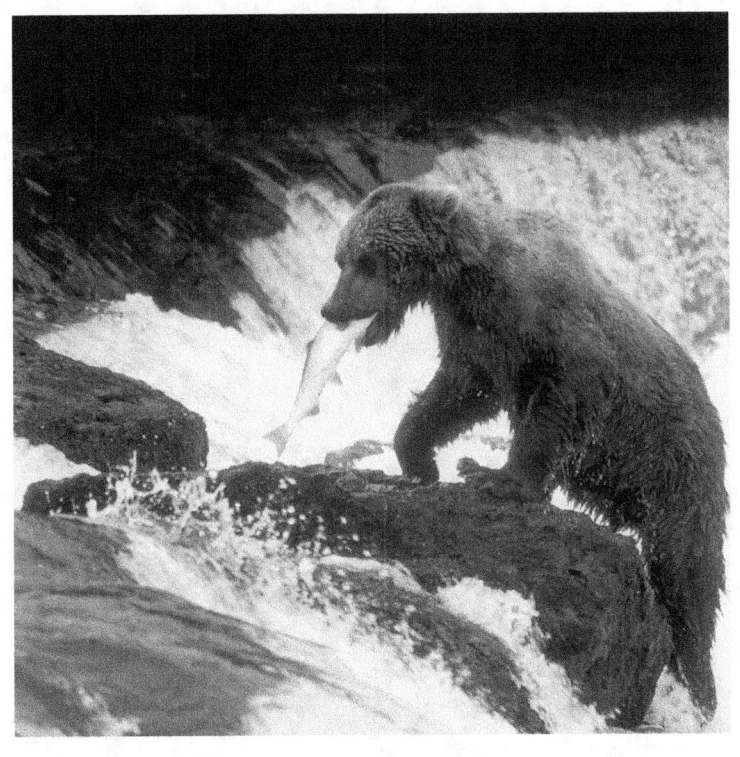

Choose wild caught fish rather than farm raised for
higher levels of Omega 3 fatty acids and less mercury

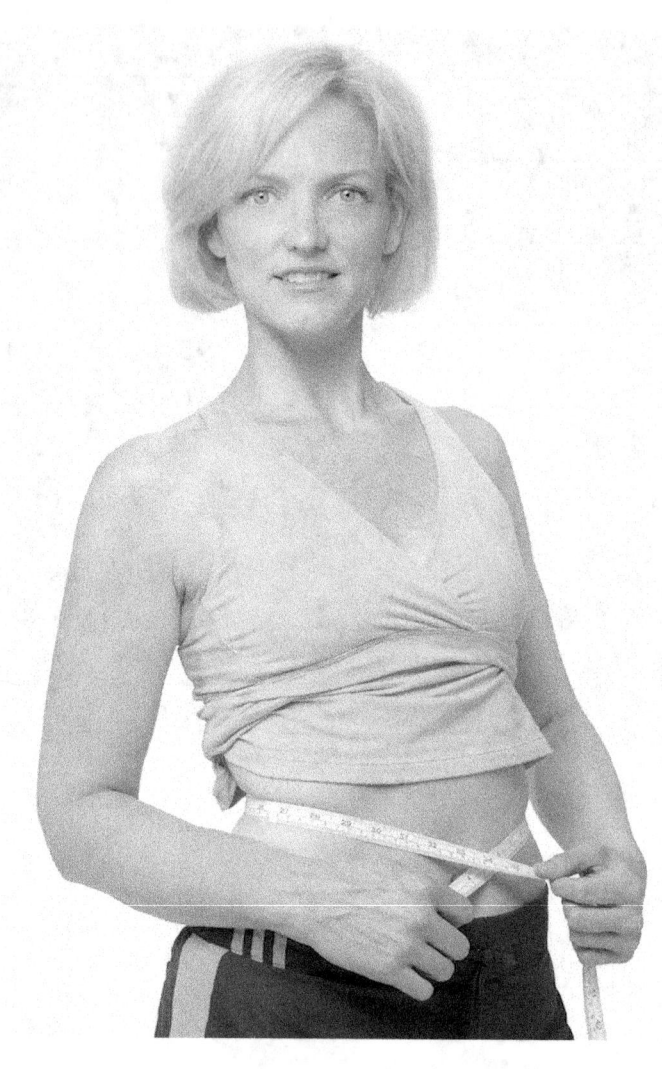

Aim for progress, not perfection

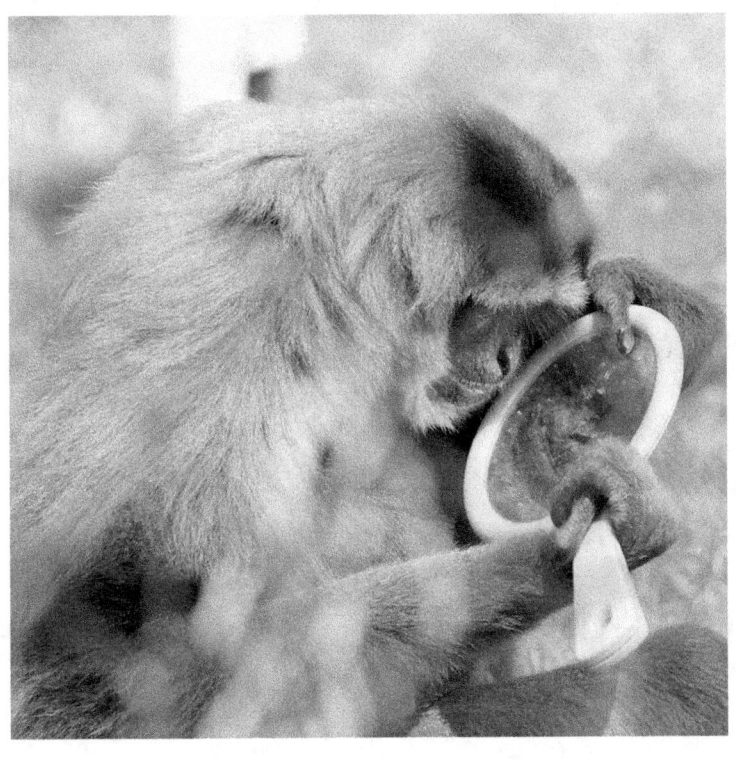

Your mirror will tell you what none of your friends will

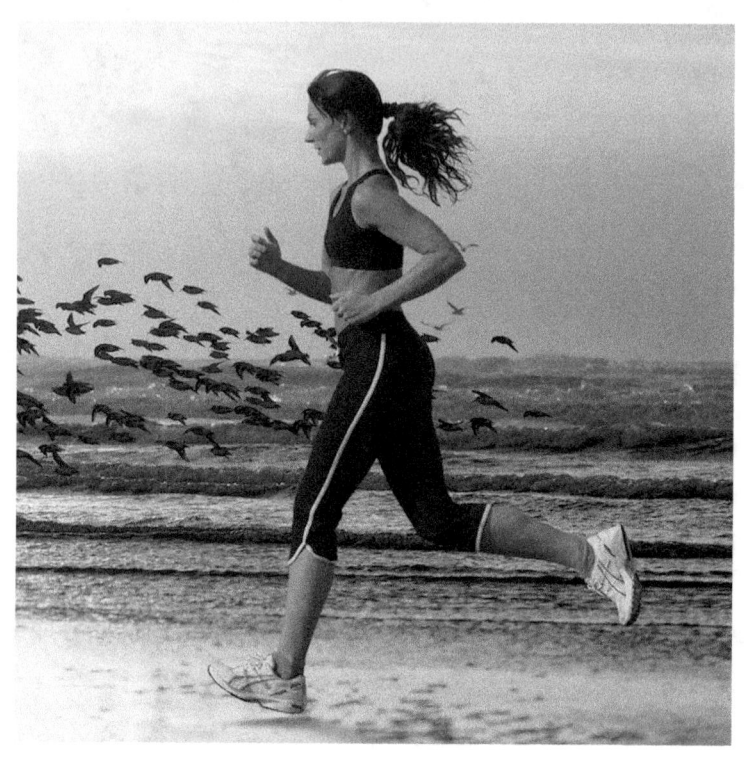

Make exercise routine, if you don't it won't happen

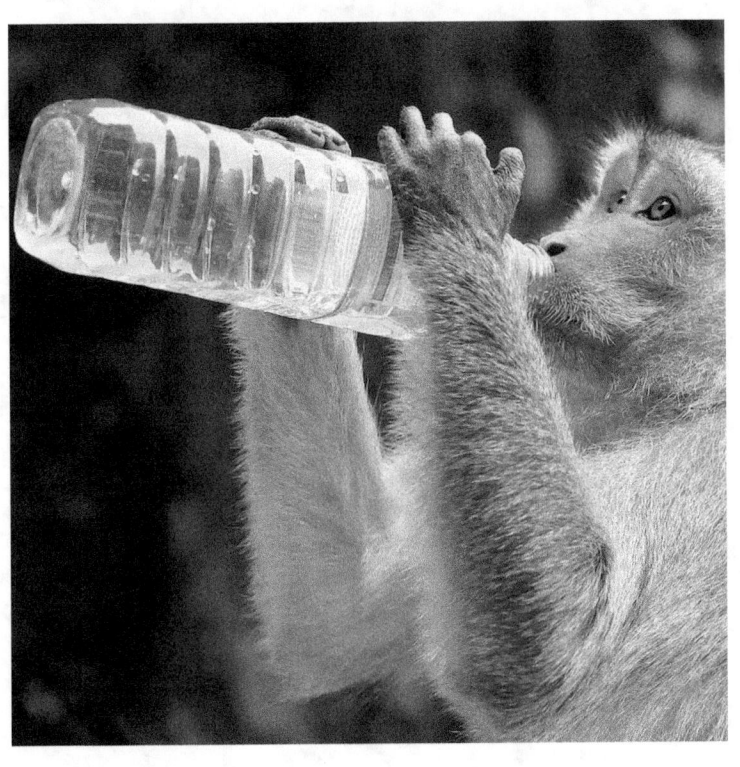

Drink plenty of water while you work out
to prevent dehydration

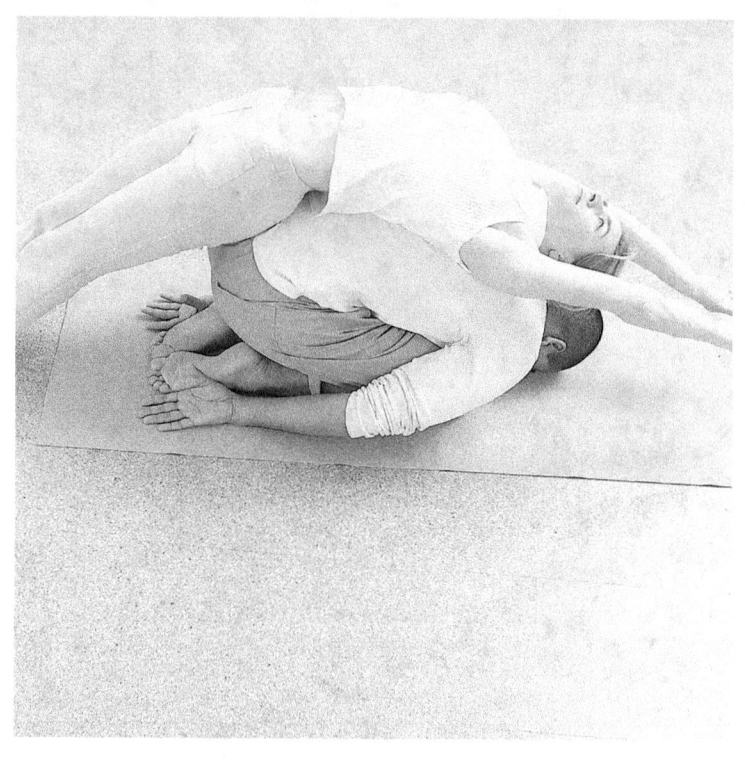

Take up yoga to de-stress, tone and improve flexibility

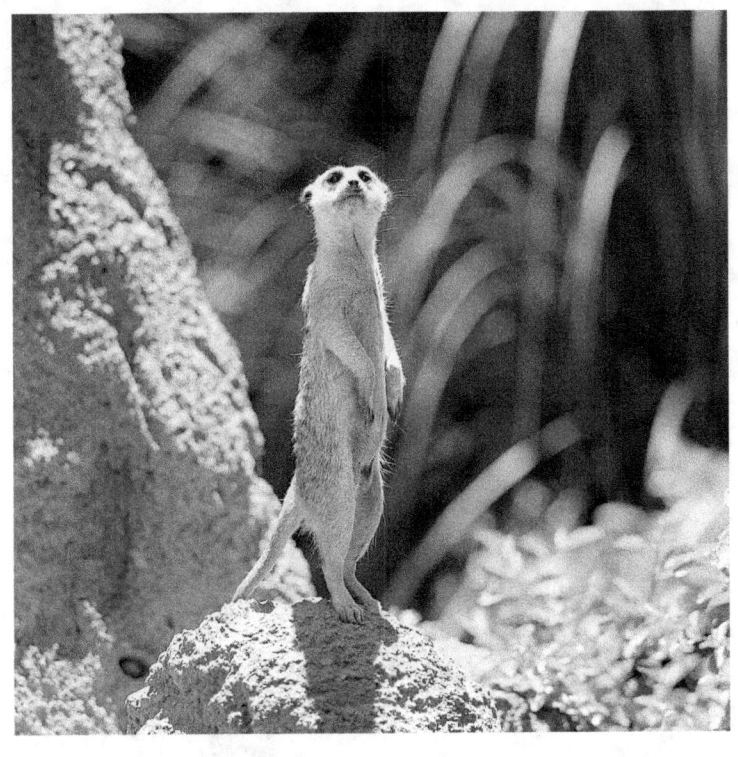

Be aware of your posture, slouching inhibits digestion

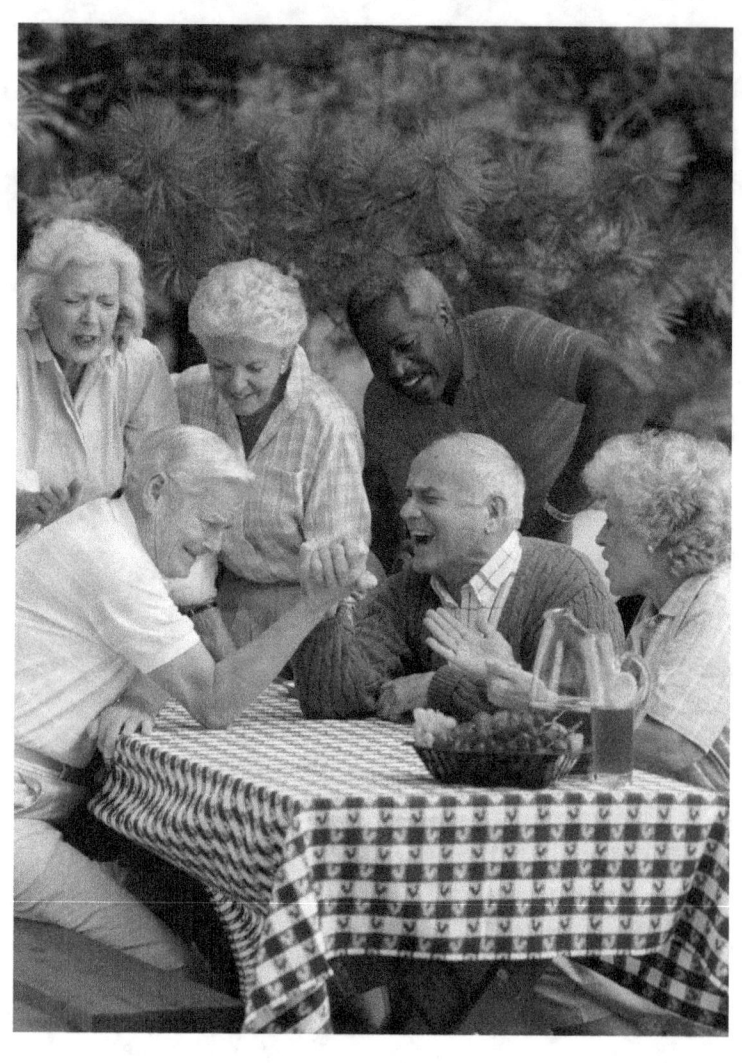

Keeping active slows the aging process

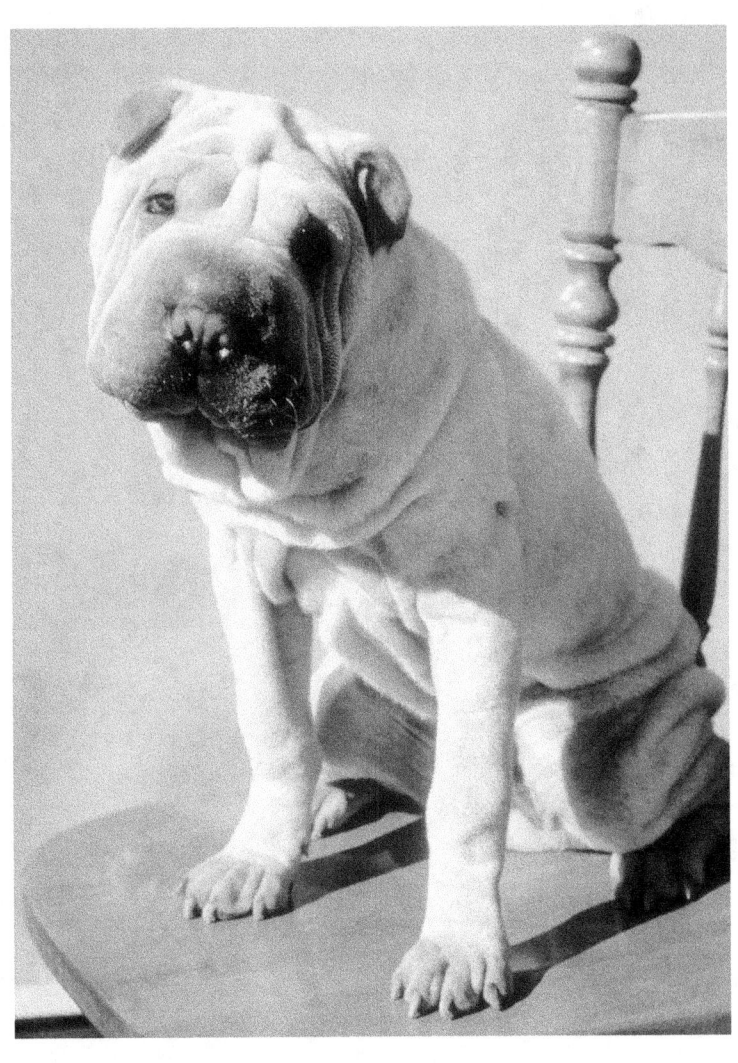

Learn to sleep on your back to prevent facial wrinkles

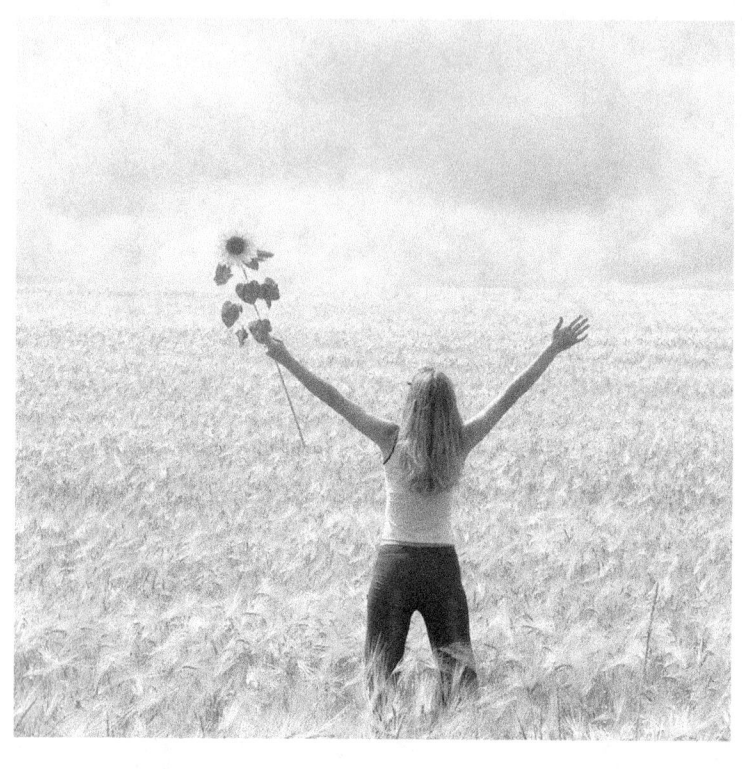

Every new day is the first day of the rest of your life and
an opportunity to start over and try again

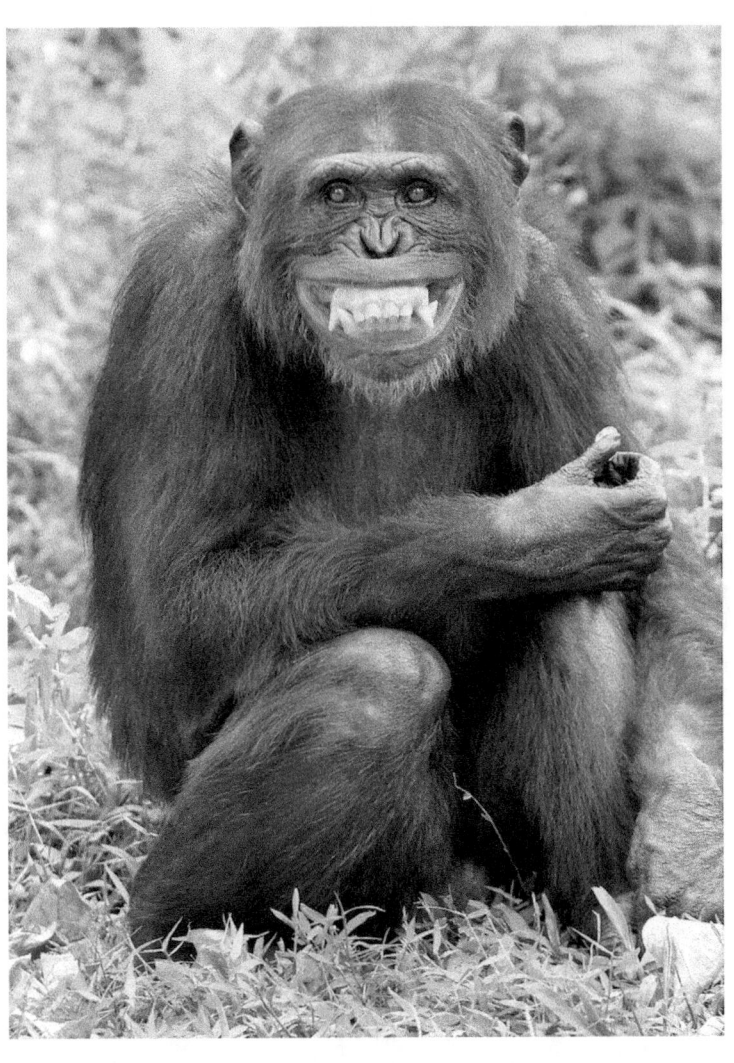

A positive attitude brings positive results

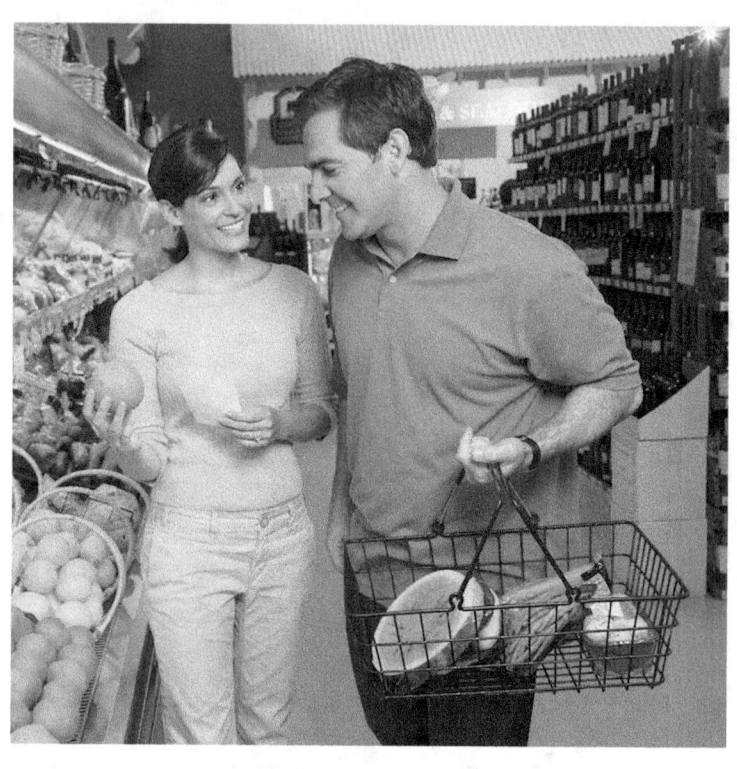

Plan you meals in advance to avoid
last minute unhealthy choices

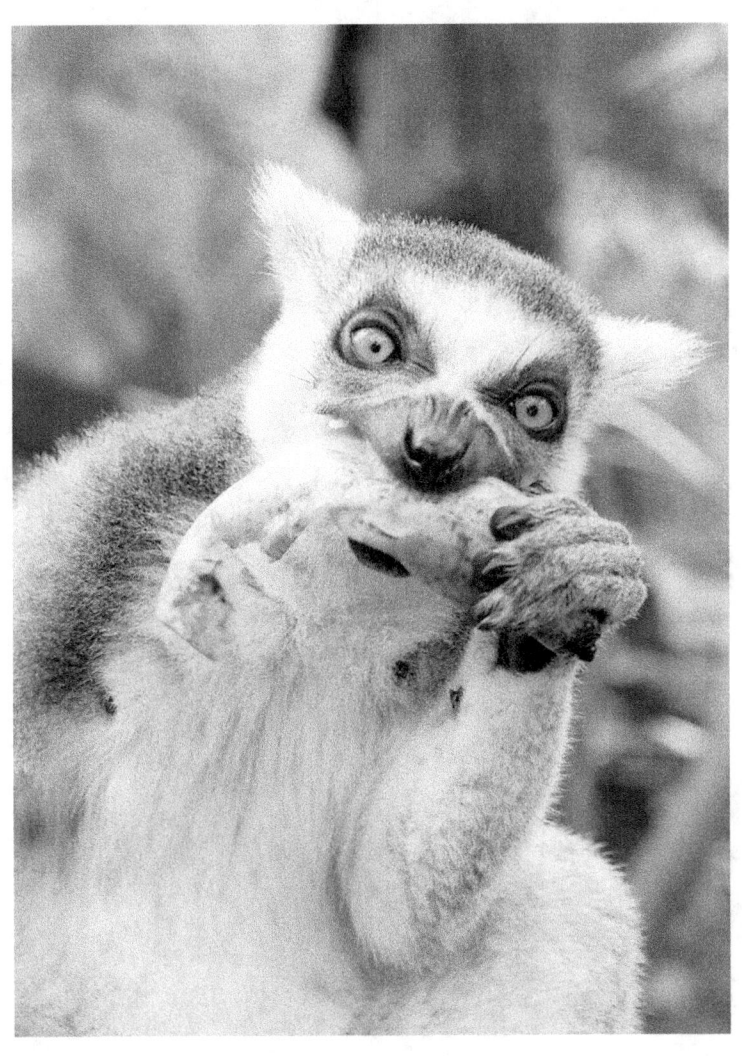

Eat fruit to satisfy a sweet tooth

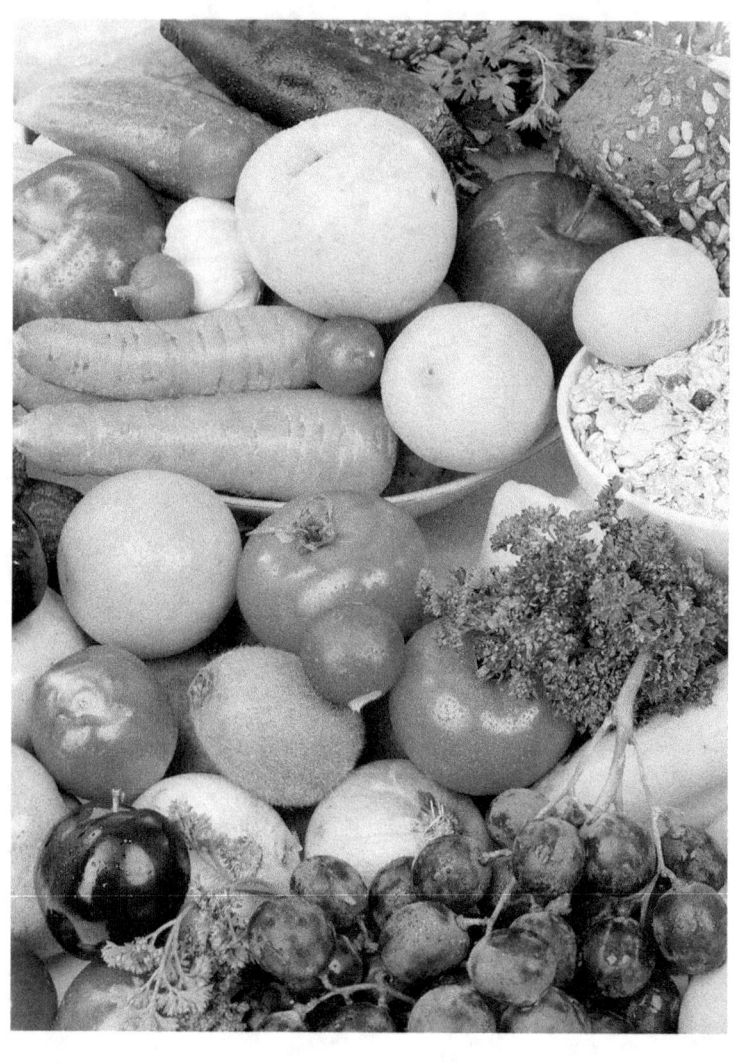

Eat foods rich in fiber to make you feel fuller for longer

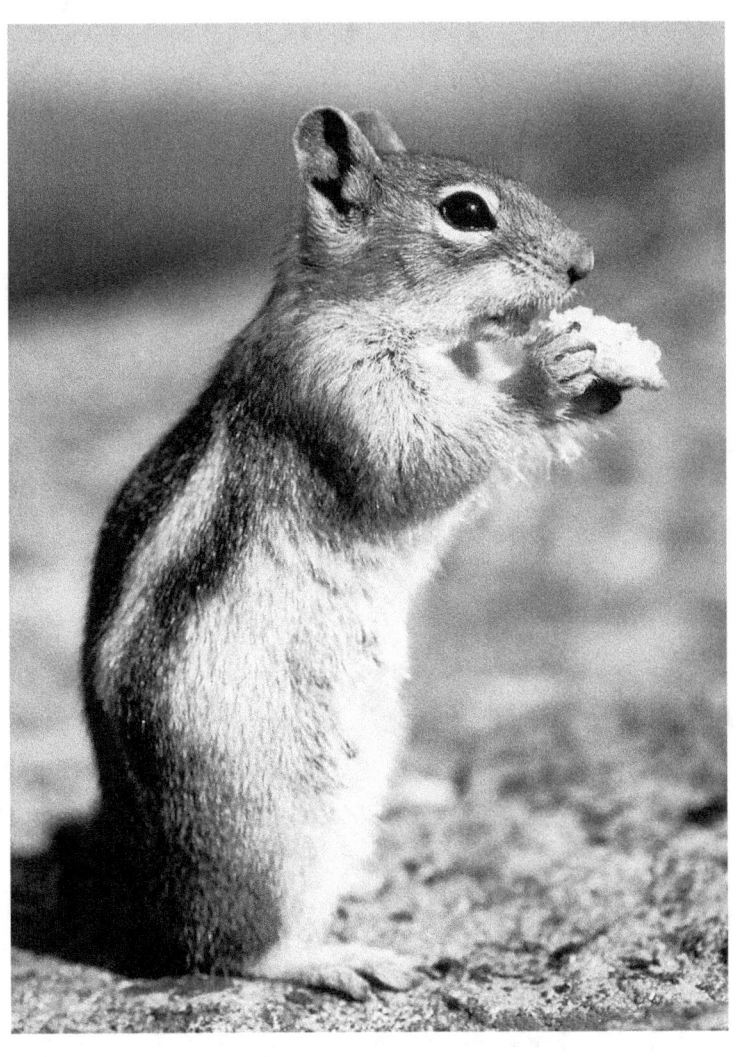

To prevent overeating, eat slowly as it takes around twenty minutes for your stomach to feel the effects of what you have already eaten

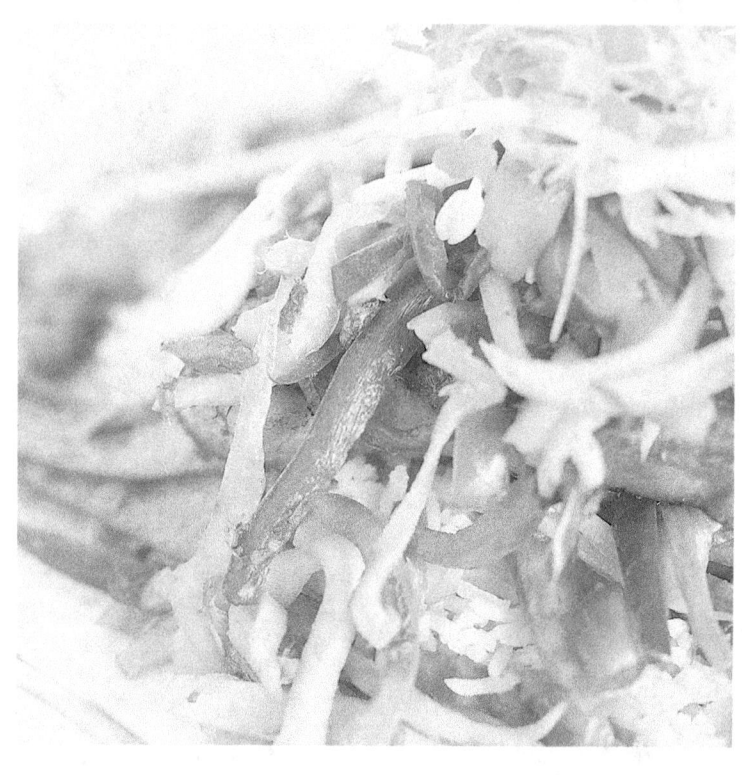

Start dinner with a salad to reduce your appetite

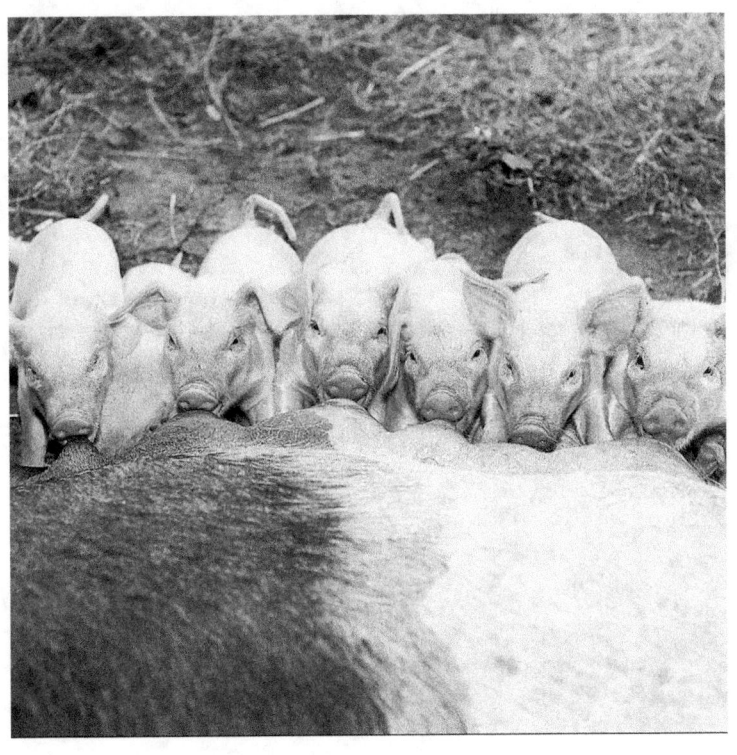

Eat as much as you need but never as much as you can

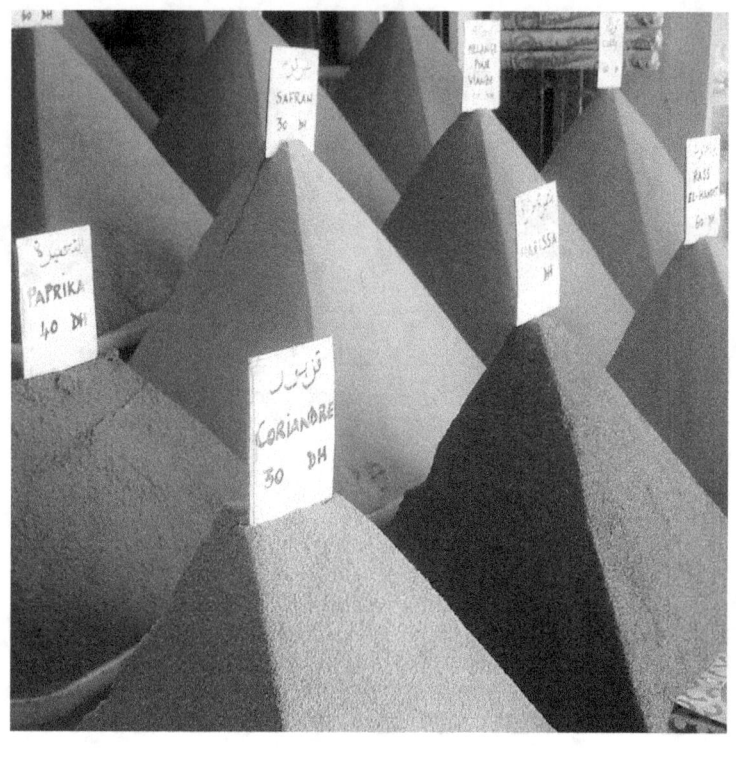

Use herbs and spices to add flavor to food
instead of fattening sauces

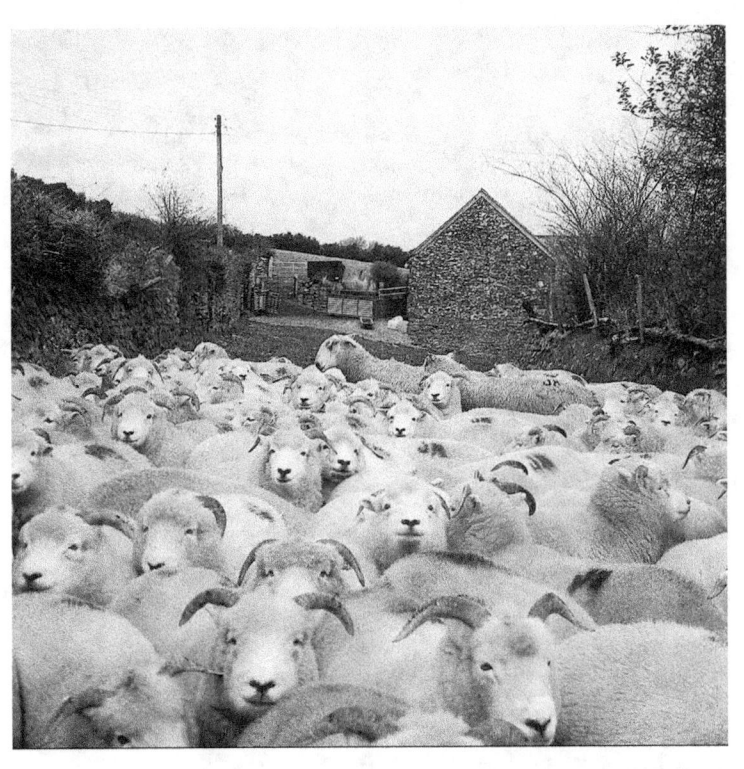

Don't follow the bad habits of others

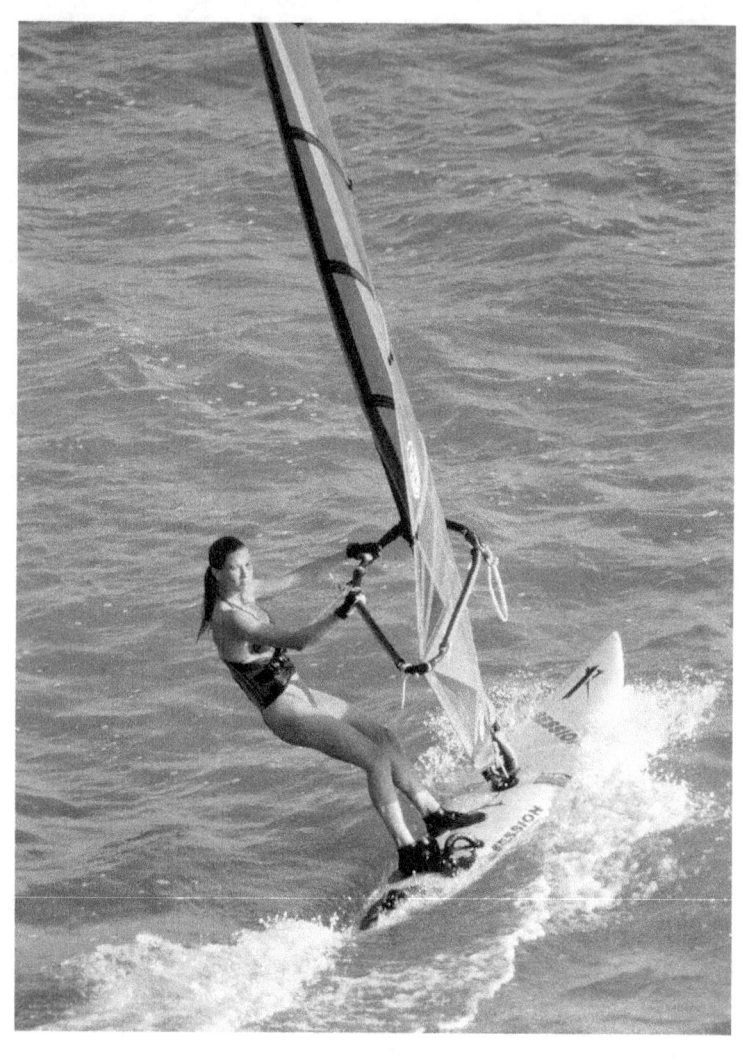

Put all your energy into living in the present moment

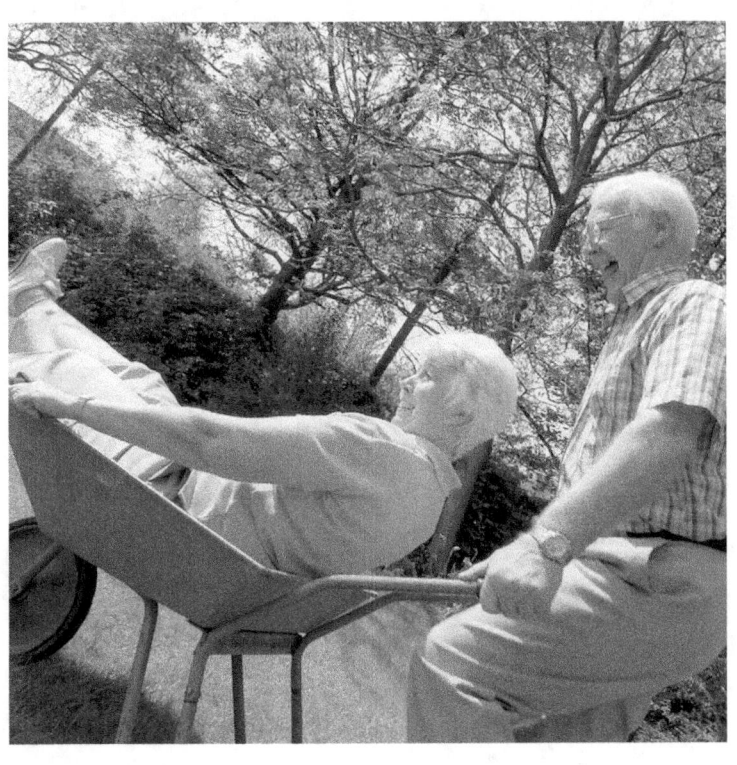

People who live long, long to live

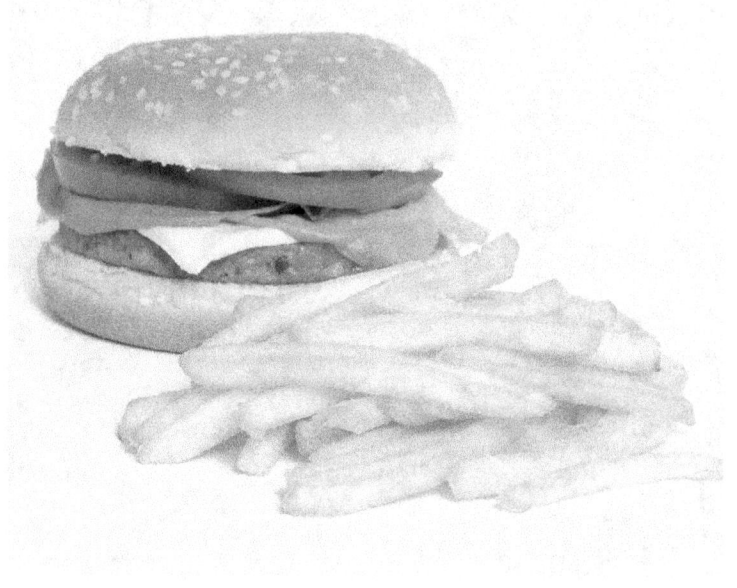

If you eat from a fast food restaurant
order the children's meal to limit calorie intake

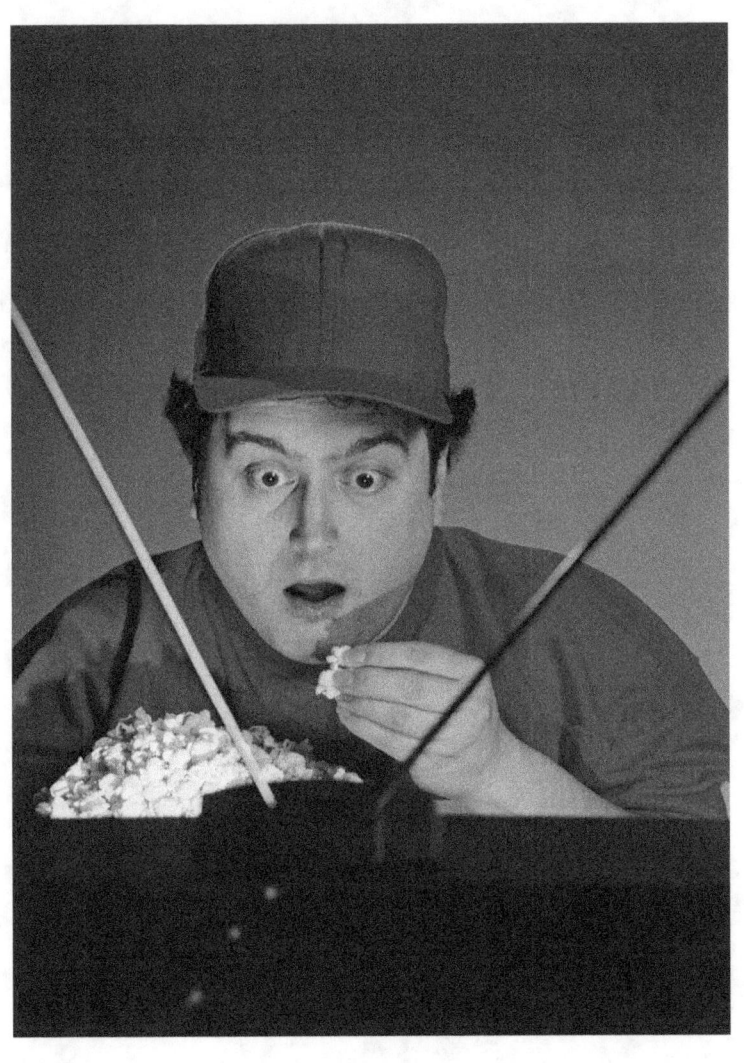

Don't eat in front of the television,
you are more likely to eat more than you need

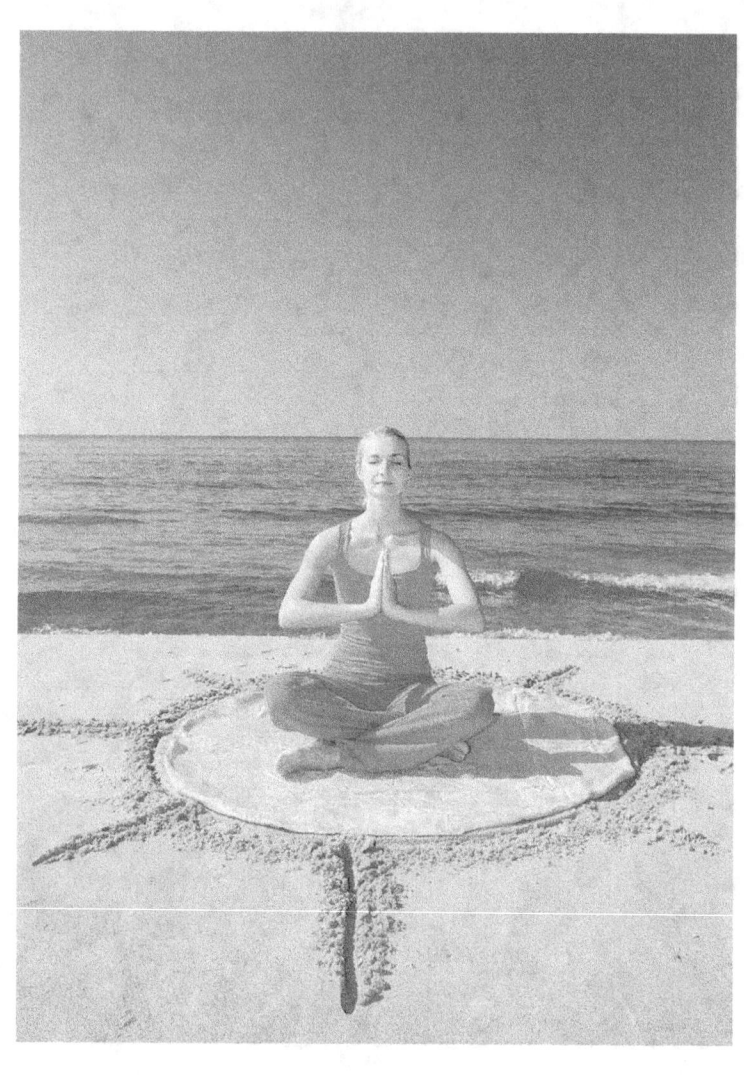

Good health begins in the mind

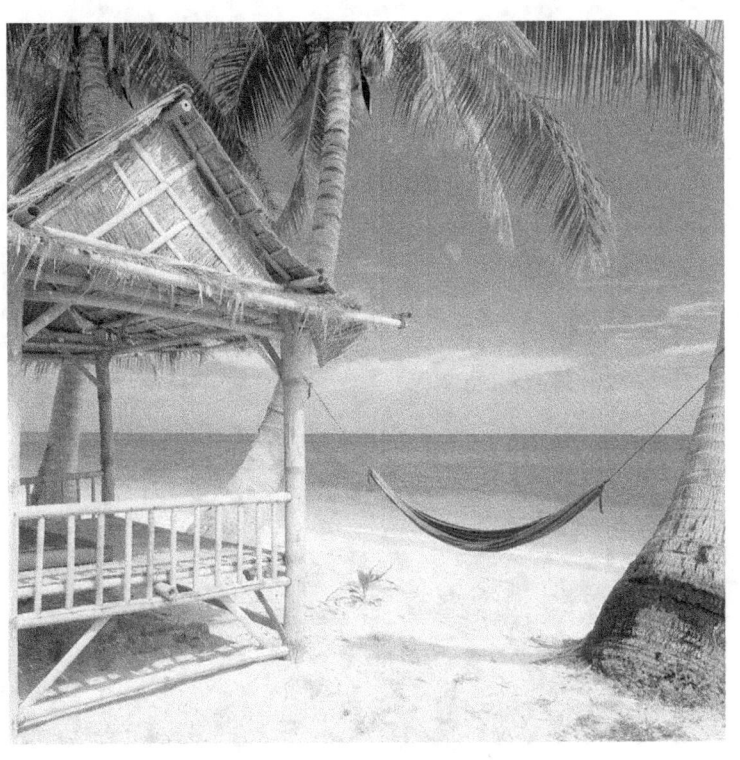

Take a vacation

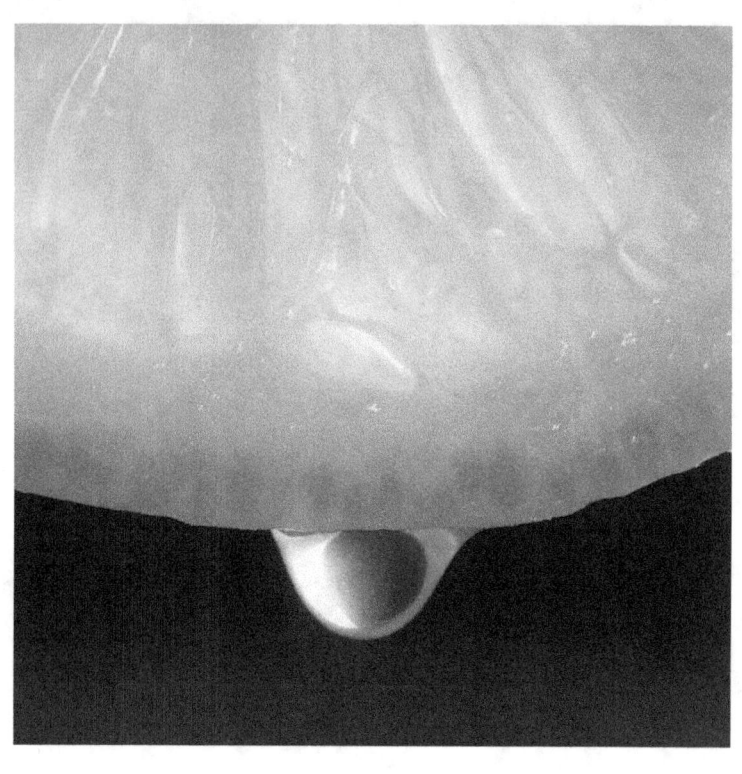

Add fresh lemon juice to vegetables instead of salt
for extra flavor

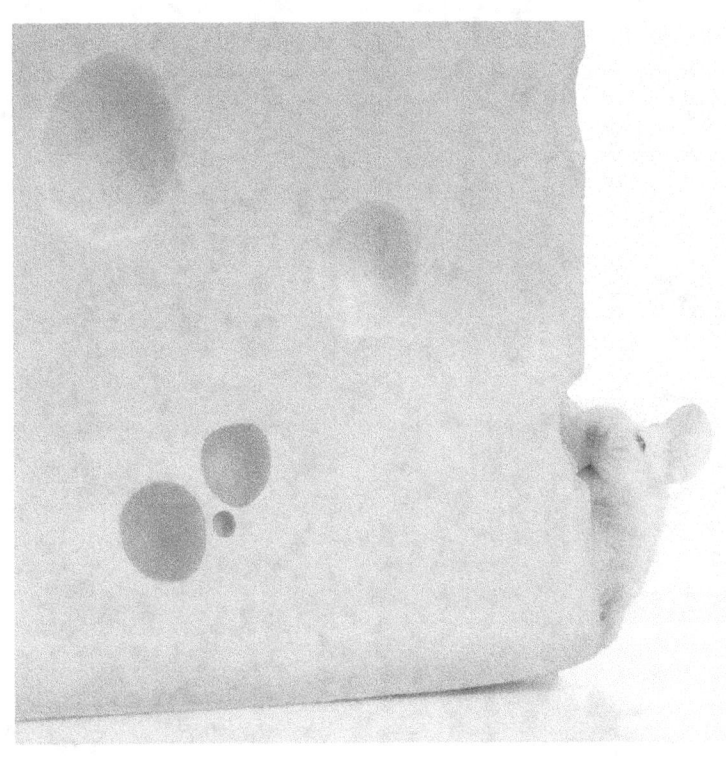

Replace regular cheese in recipes with a smaller
amount of a more flavorful cheese

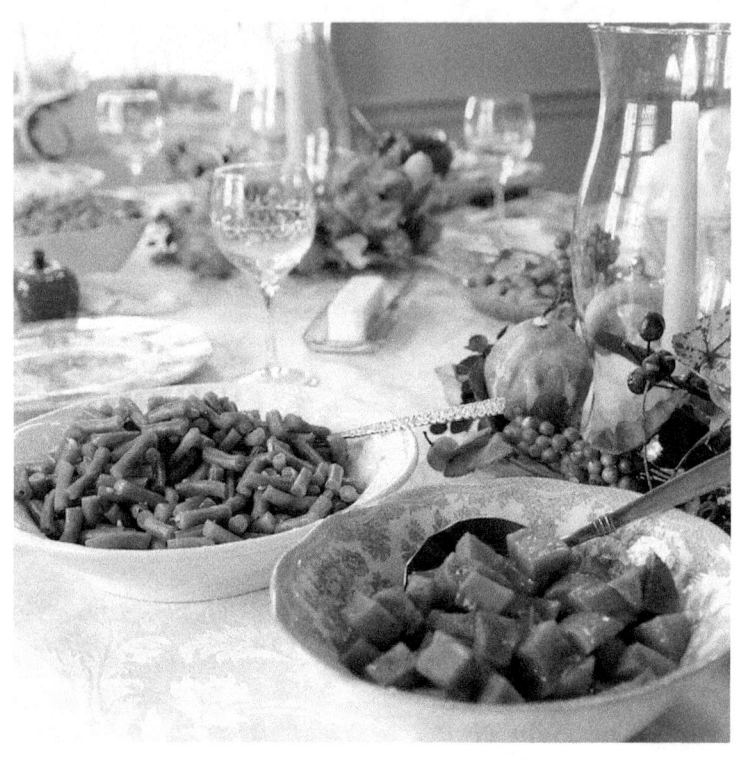

If you plan on going to an event where you will eat more than usual, minimize calories during the rest of the day

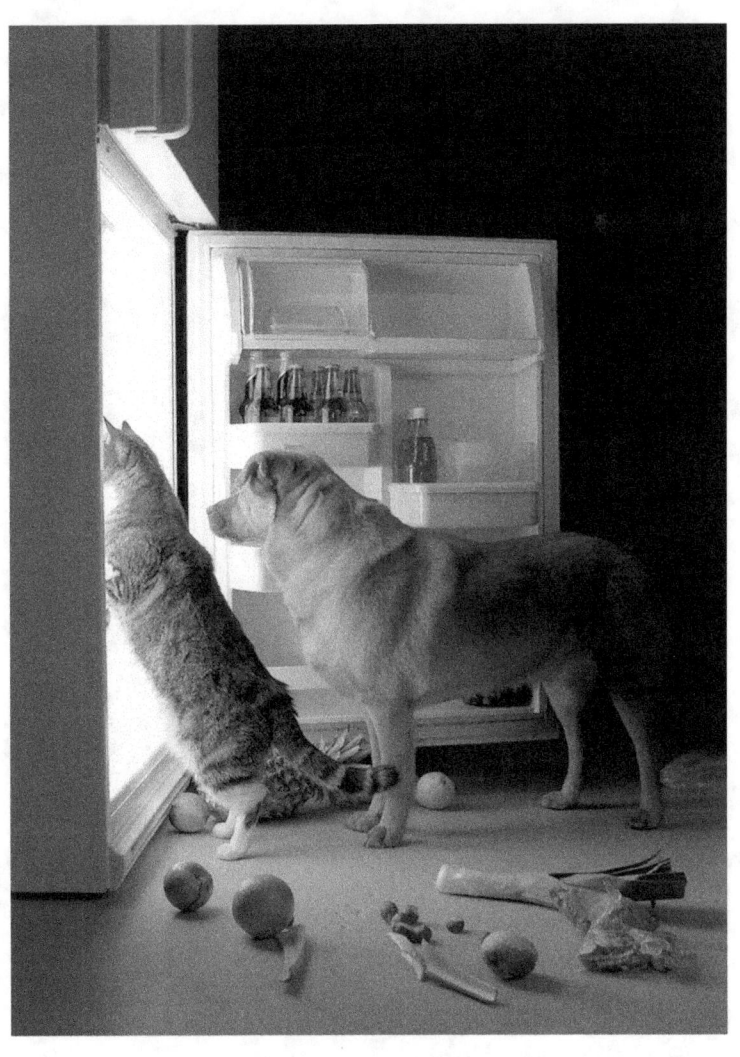

When you feel upset, tired or stressed,
stay away from the refrigerator

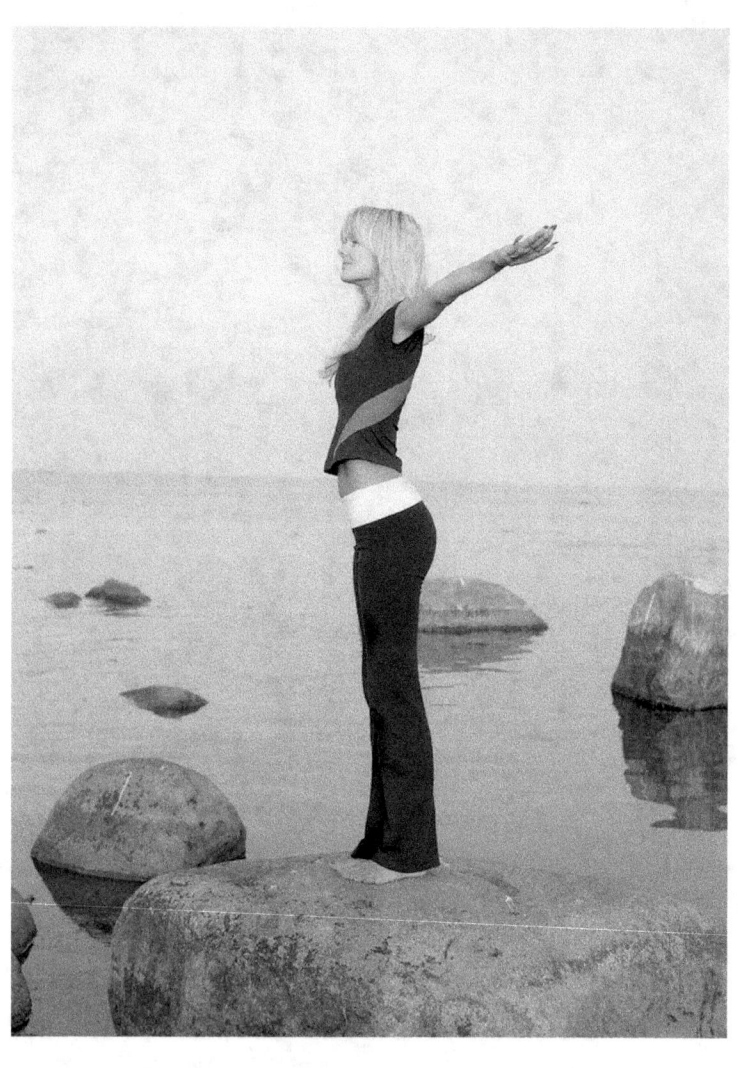

Drop self critical thoughts and be grateful for your body

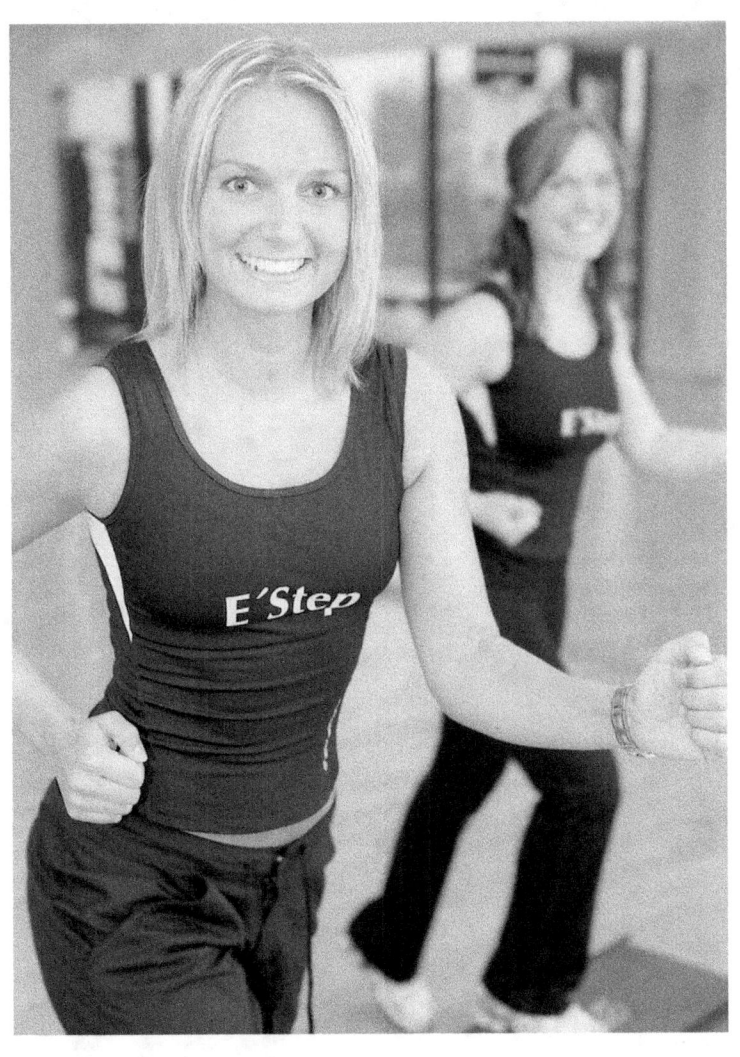

You cannot alter your body type but you can be
the best you through diet and exercise

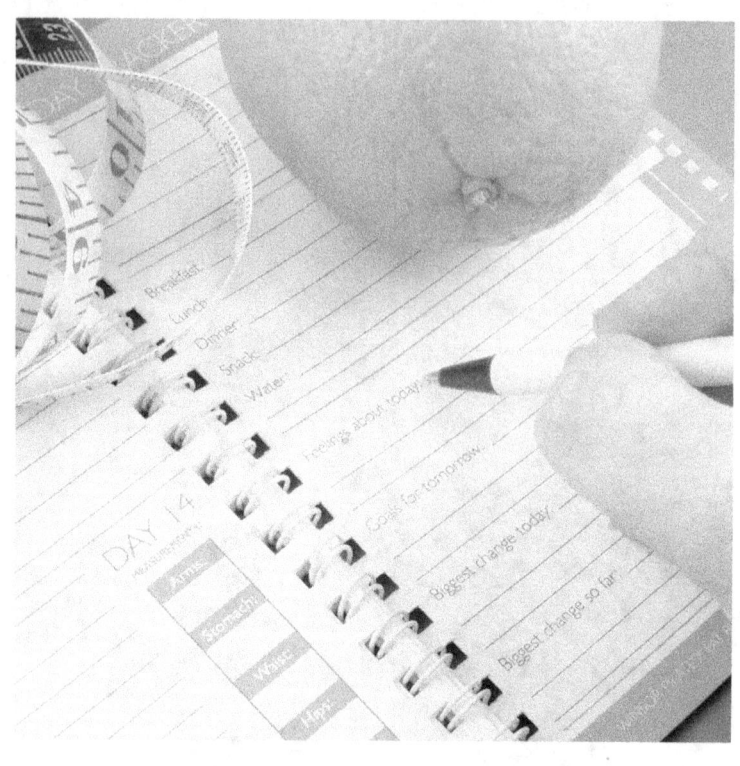

When weight training, log your progress to encourage
yourself to push to the next level

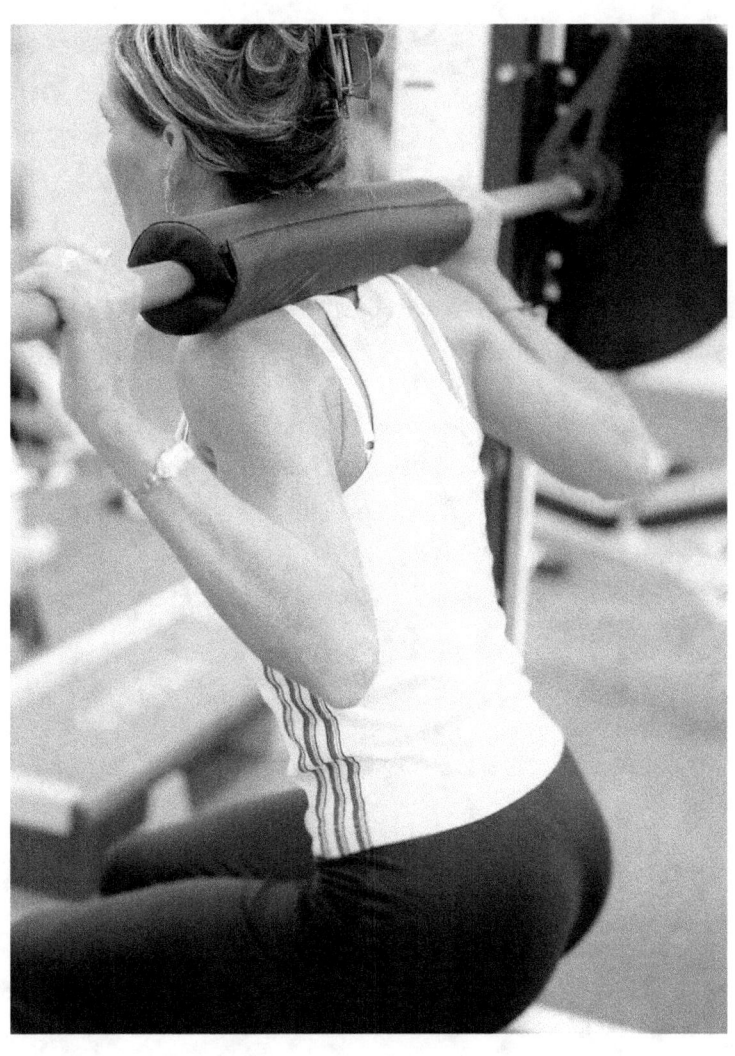

Squats and lunges are the best exercises to tone your glutes

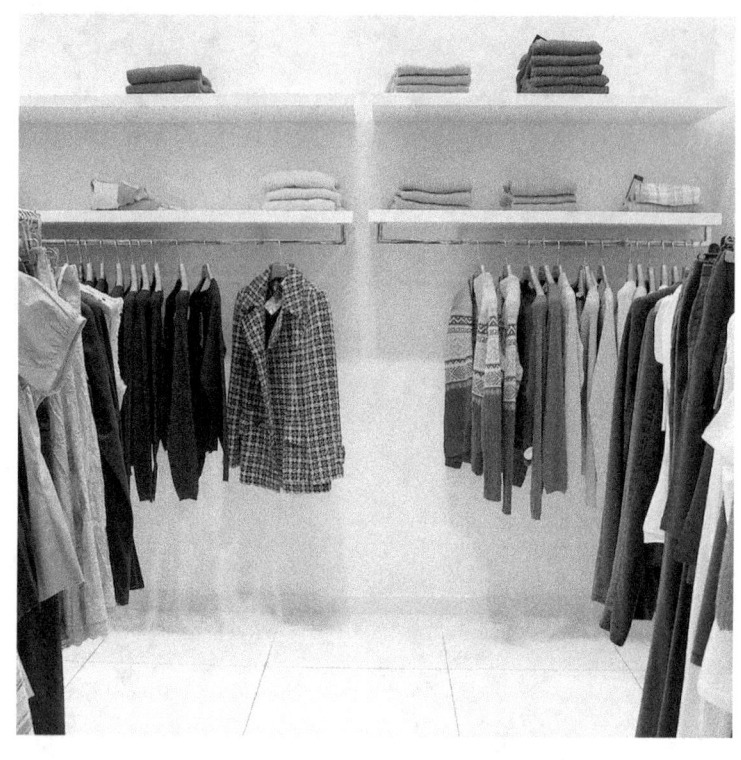

Maintaining your weight will save you money, reducing the need for different sizes of clothes in your wardrobe

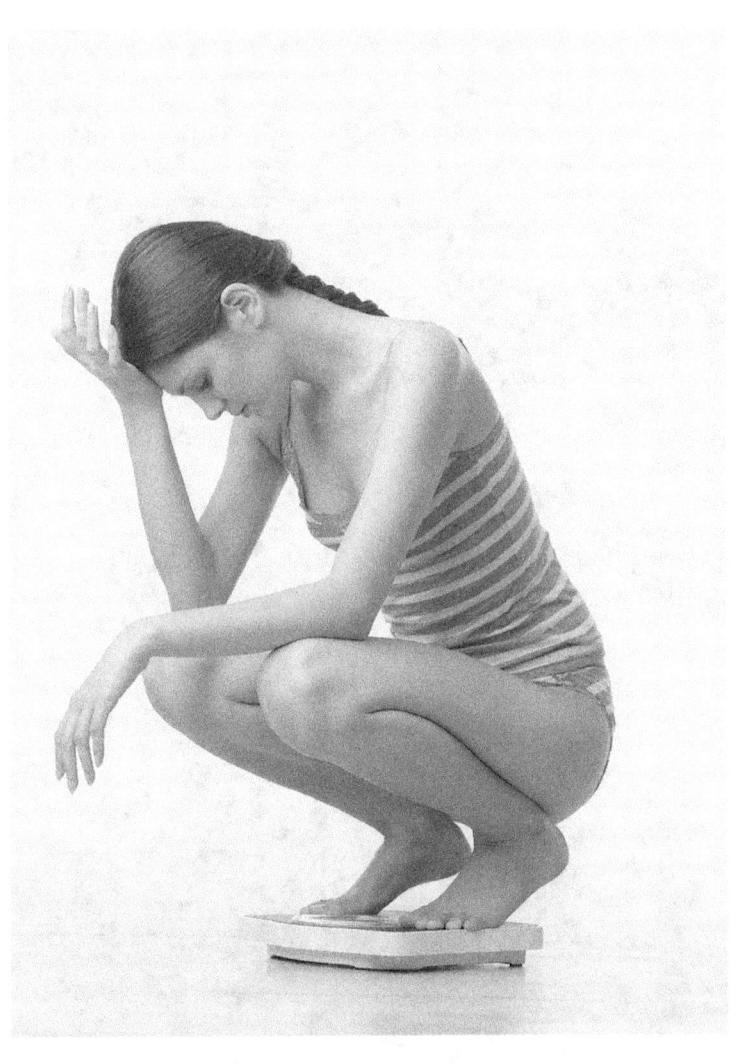

Don't weigh yourself every day

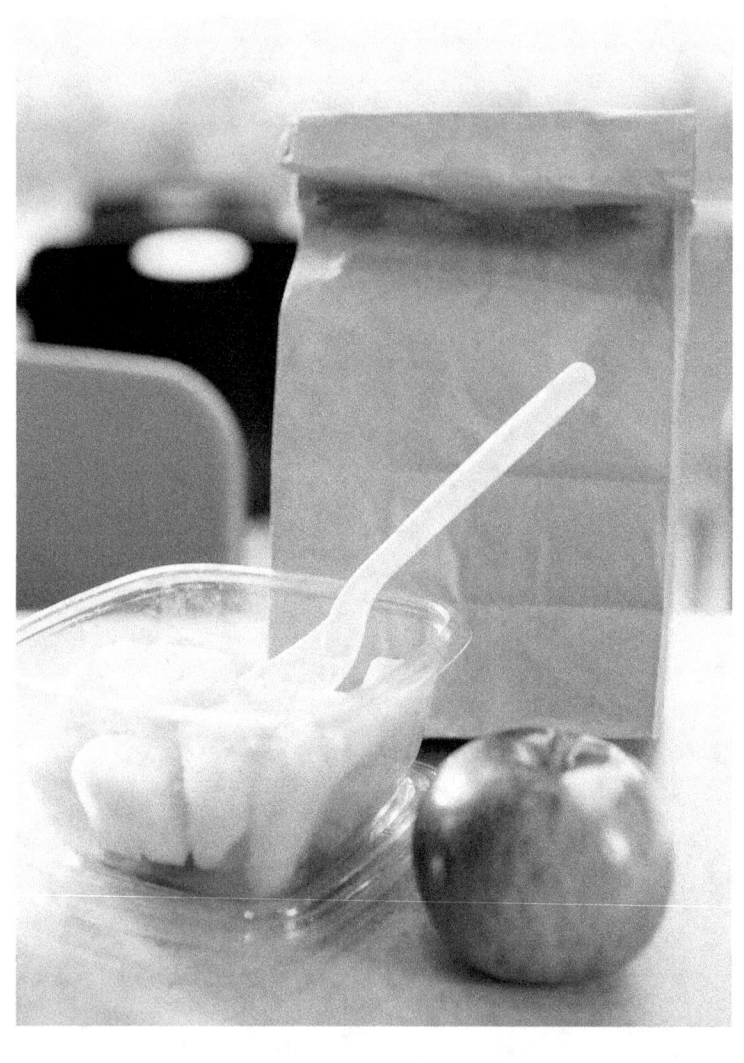

Pack your own lunches to take more control
over your daily calorie intake

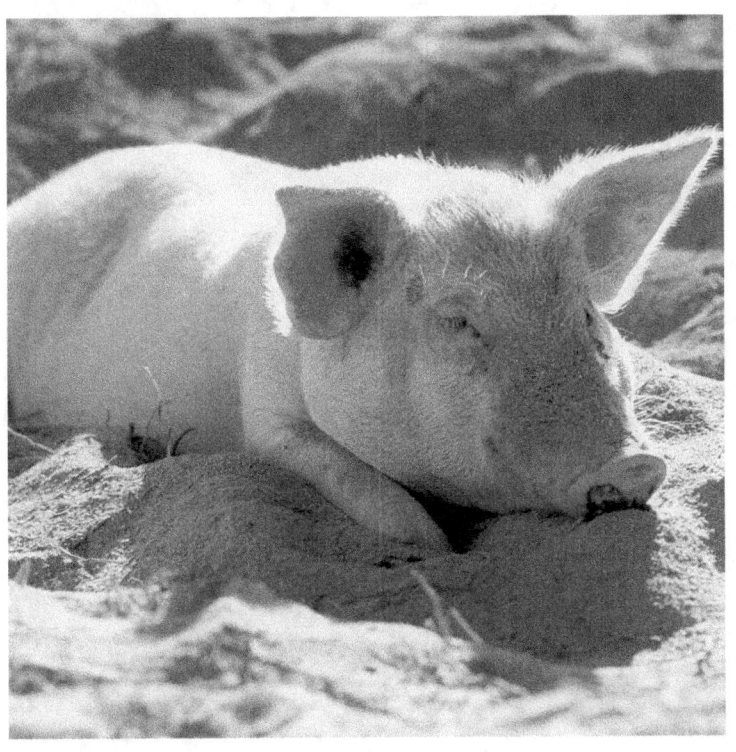

Don't skip meals, it can cause you to overeat later in the day

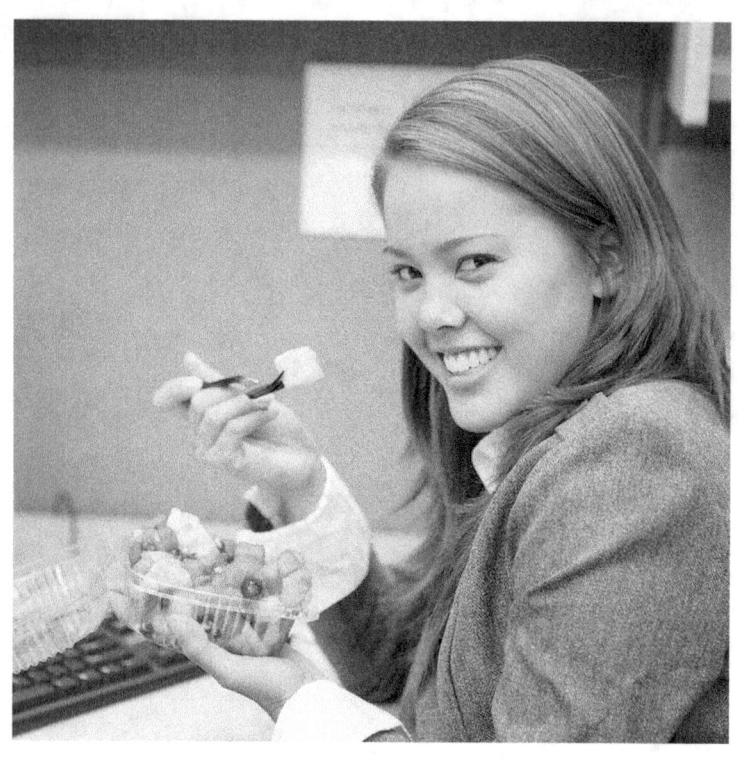

Take healthy snacks to work to reduce your chances of
visiting the vending machine

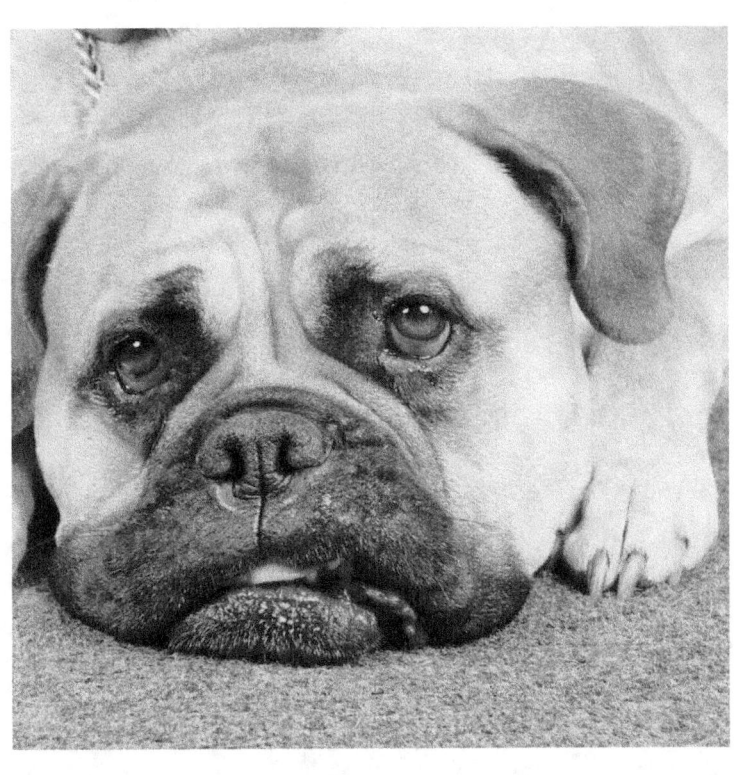

Don't eat just to fight tiredness

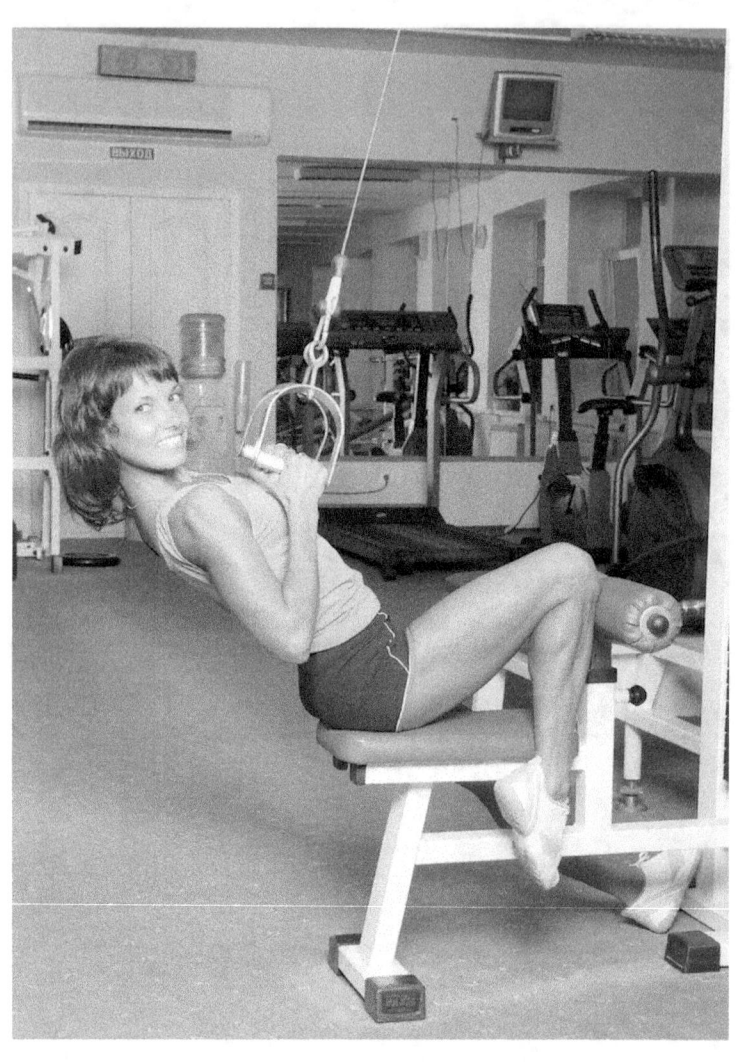

If you want to be toned and lean, do a combination of both
weight training and aerobics at least three times a week

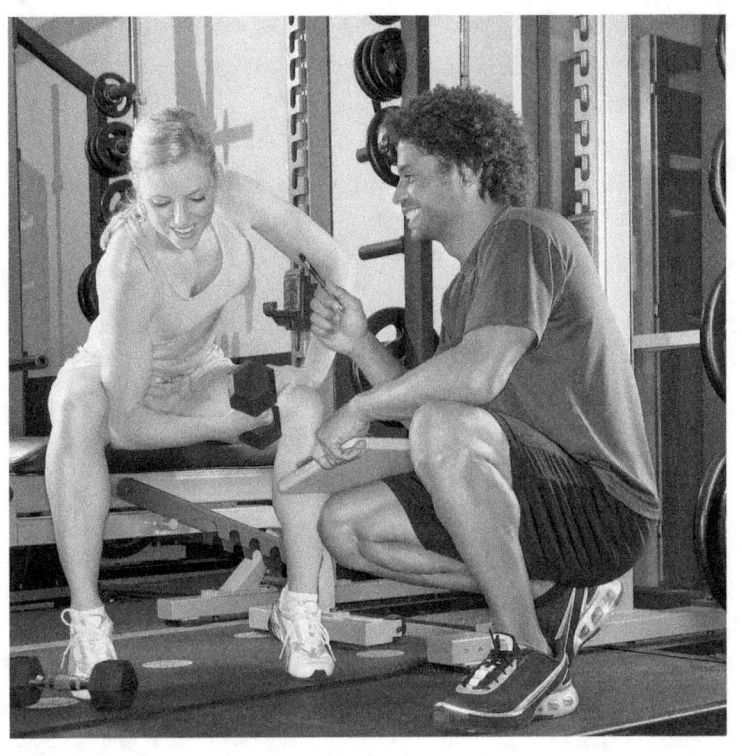

Hire a personal trainer for extra motivation

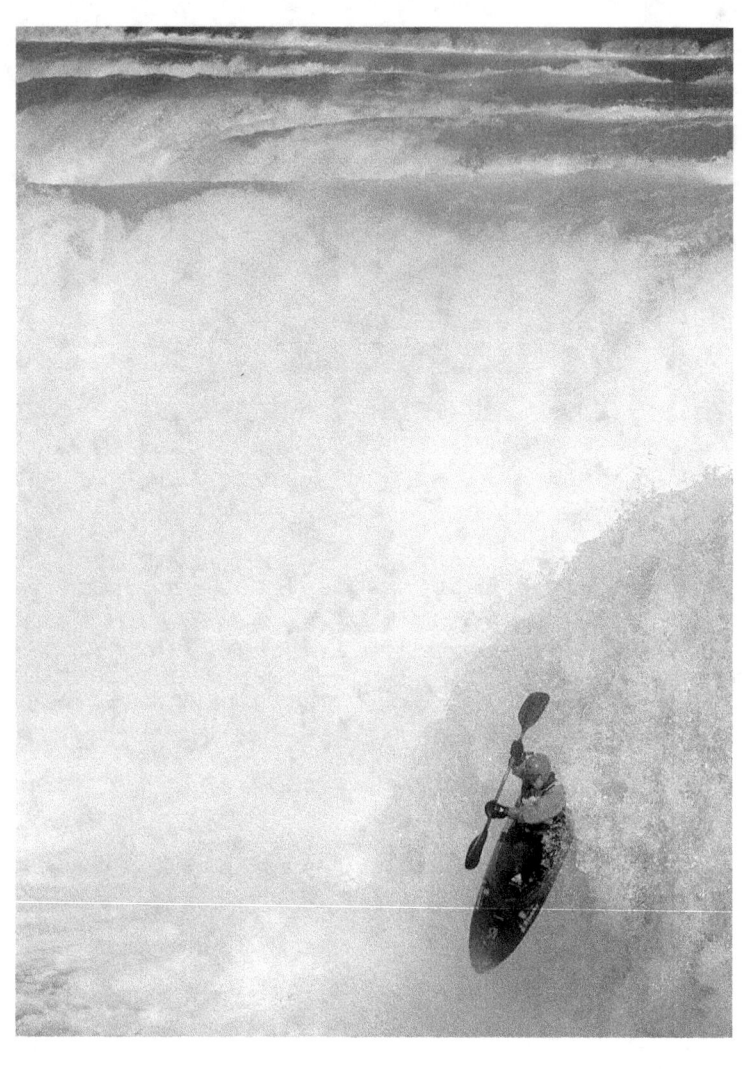

Find inspiration in others

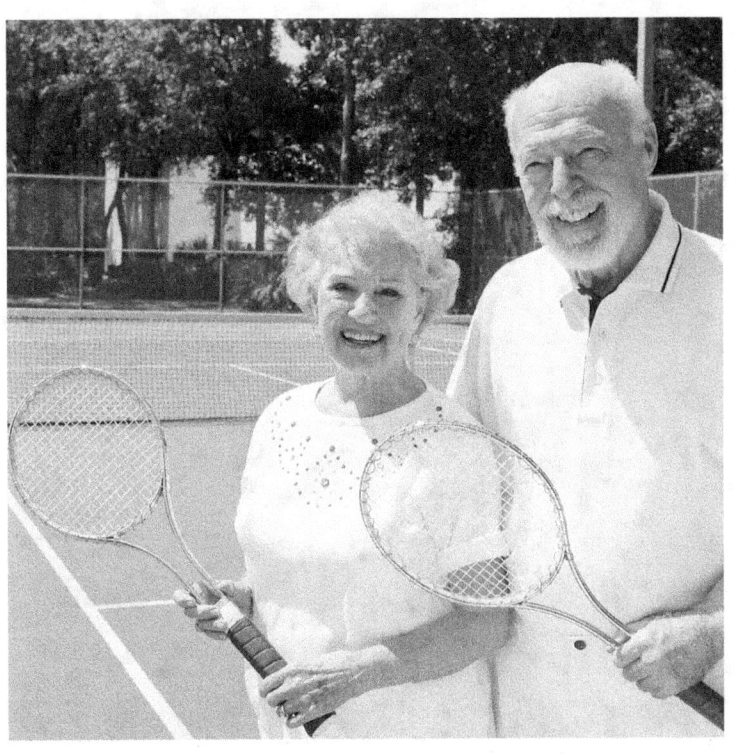

Its never too late to start over

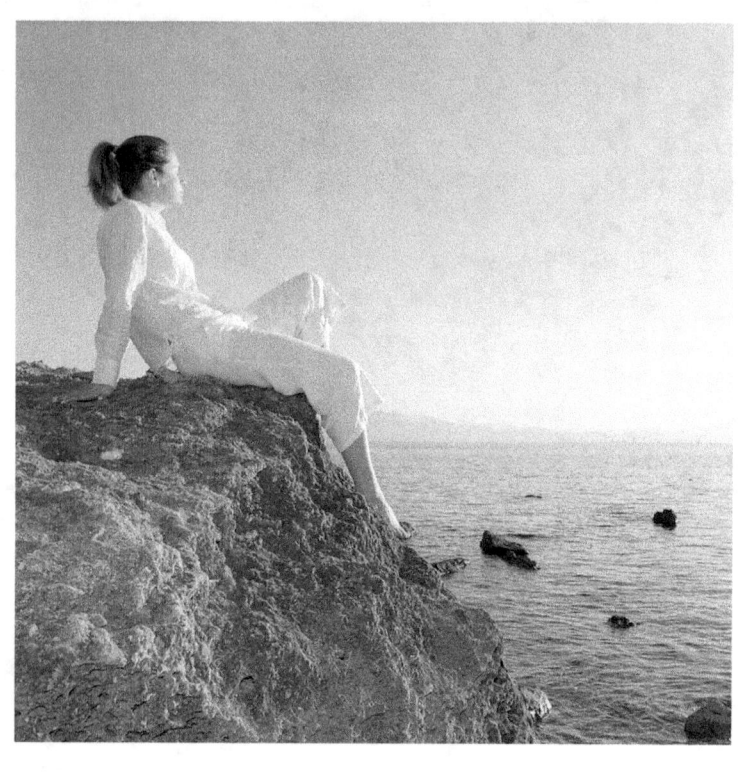

When you feel like life is passing you by in a rush,
find quiet time to reflect

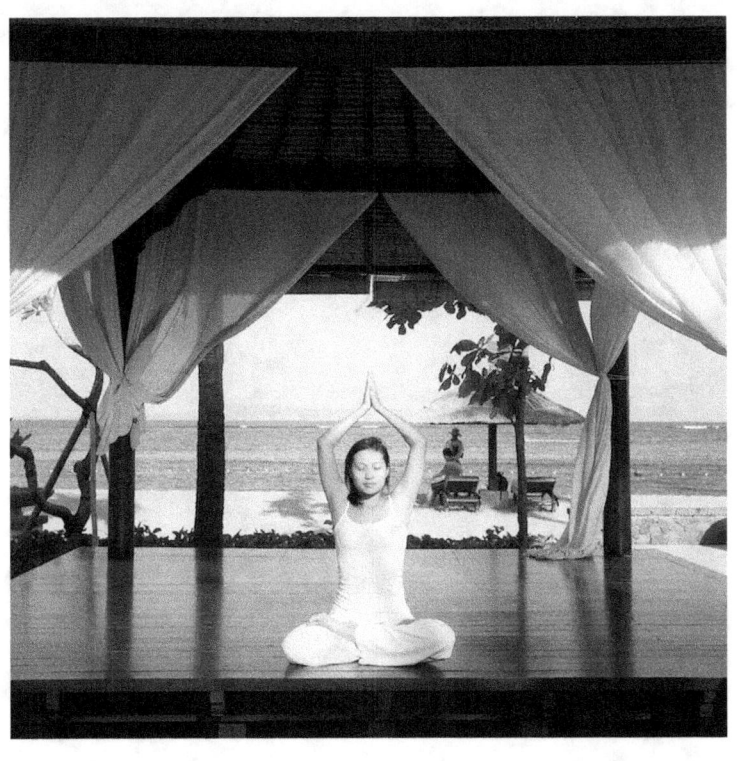

Try meditation to relax and quiet your mind

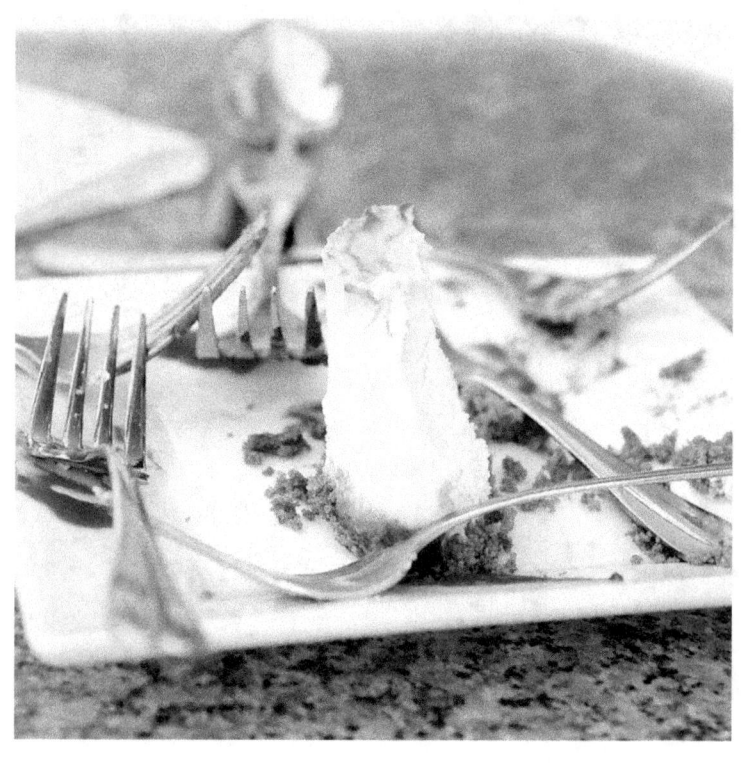

If you really want dessert, share it with friends

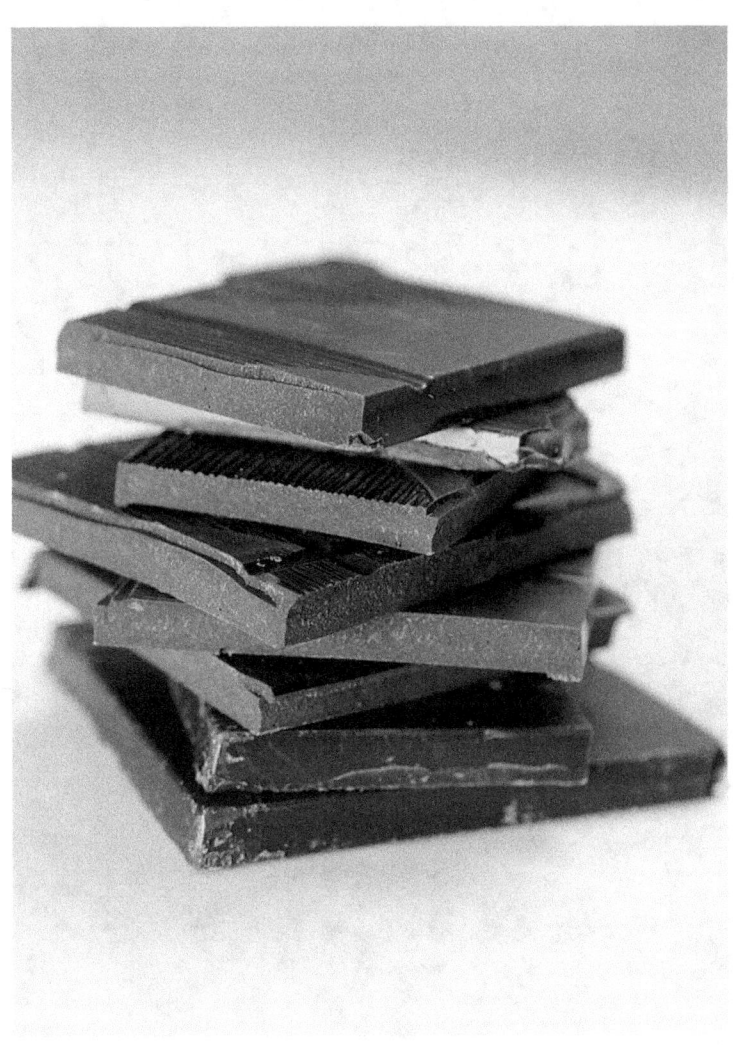

Eat a small amount of dark chocolate each day to increase
your intake of antioxidants and reduce blood pressure,
dark chocolate also has less fat than other varieties

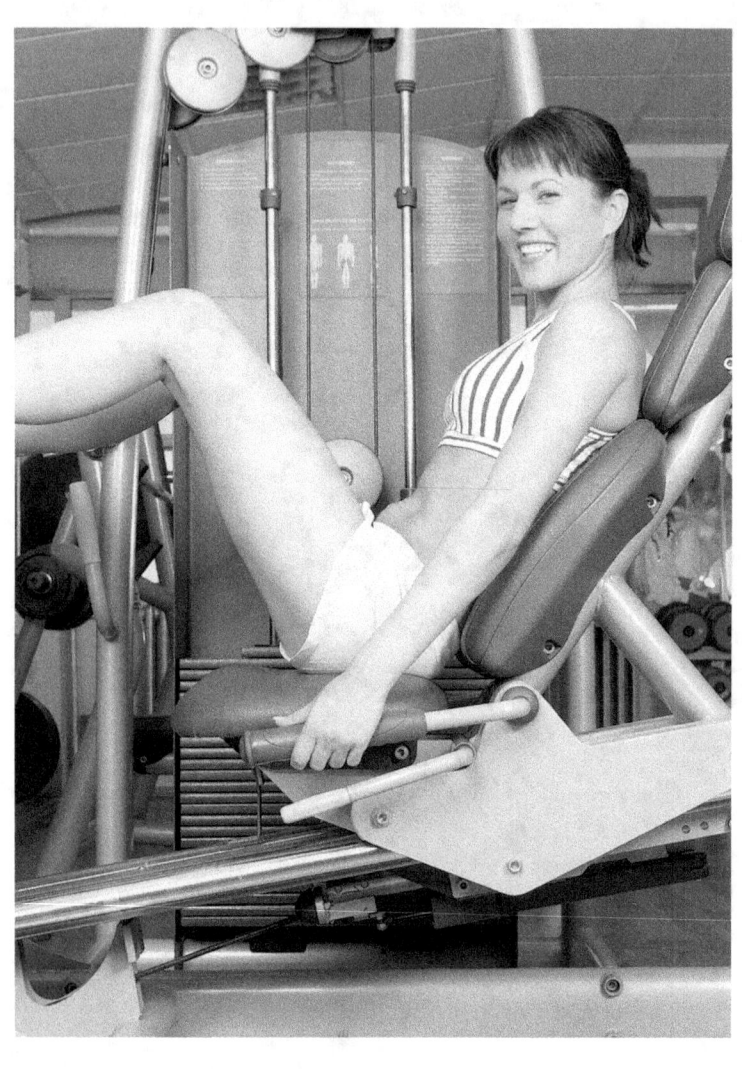

Alternate your workout routine to keep it
interesting and motivating

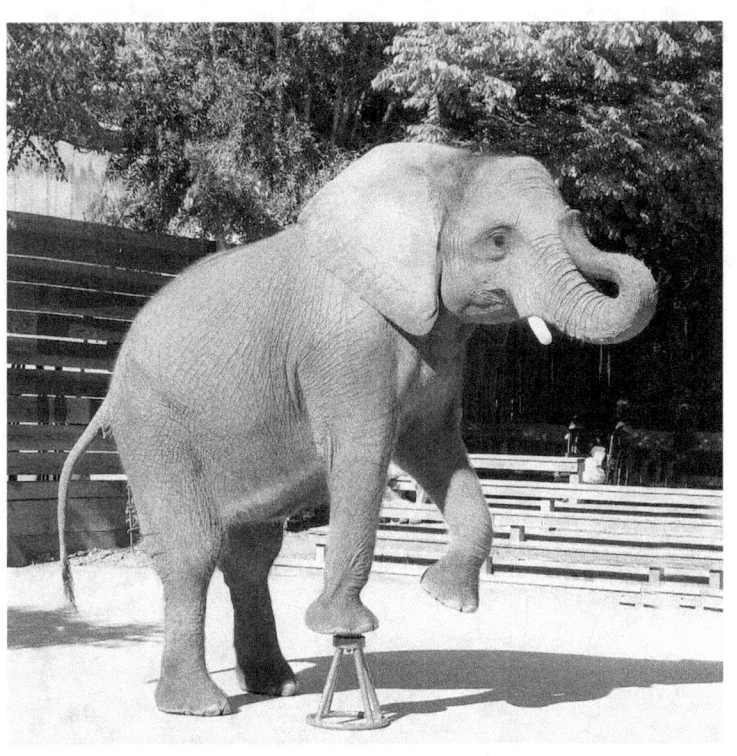

Every big change starts with a small step

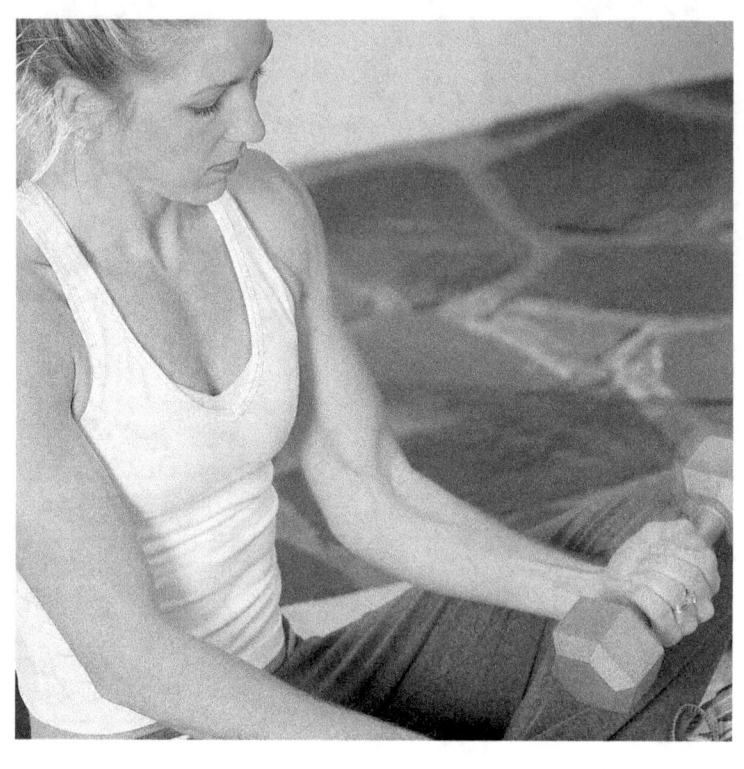

If you don't want to join a gym, buy some free weights
or a treadmill to use at home

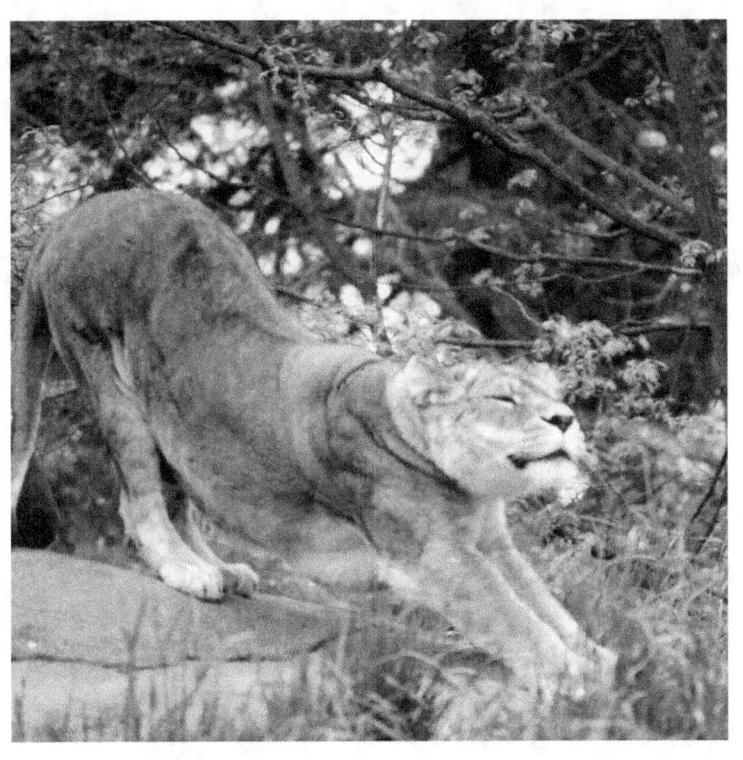

Stretch before exercising to prevent injury

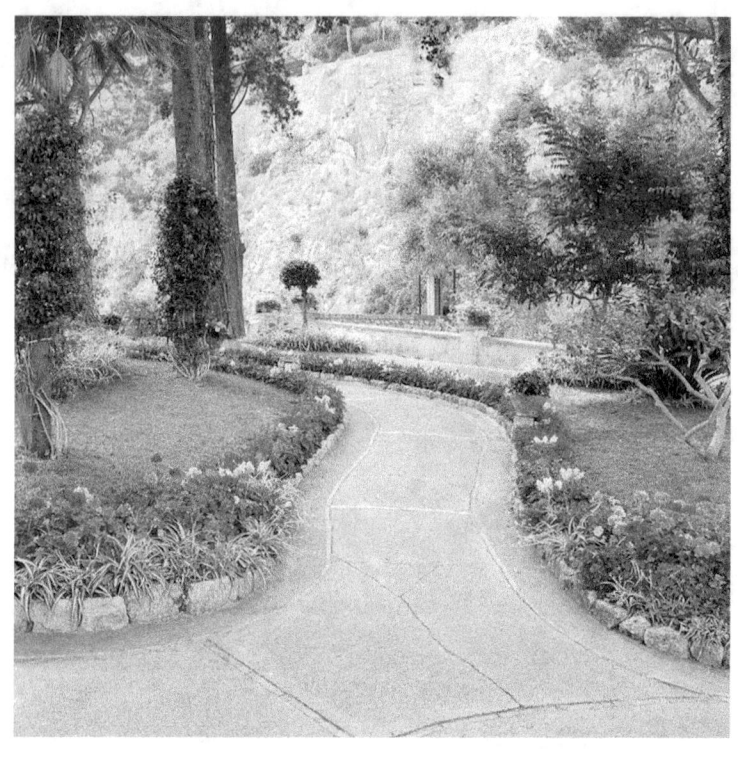

Take a walk in a park to wind down and clear your mind

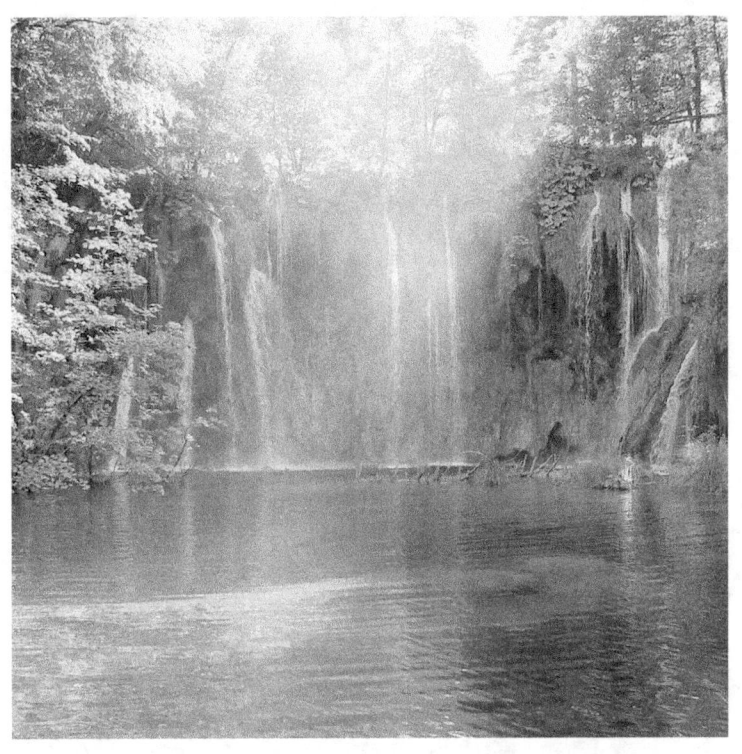

Mother nature offers the best medicine for your soul

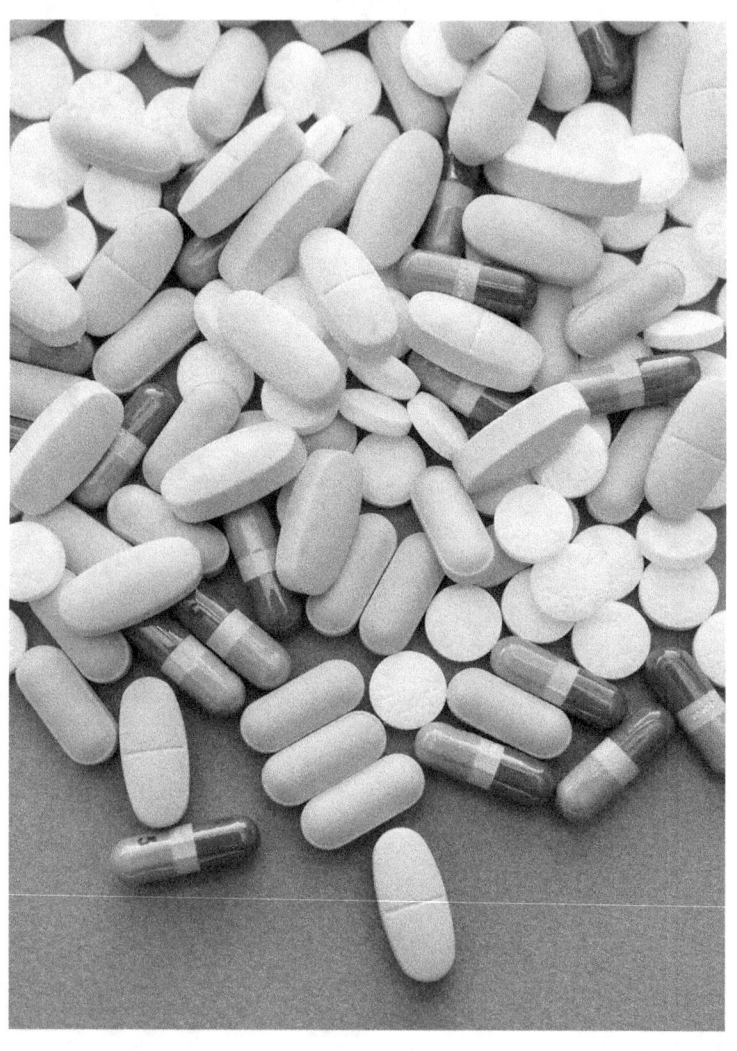

Avoid diet pills, they are no substitute for changing your behavior and can often produce undesirable side effects

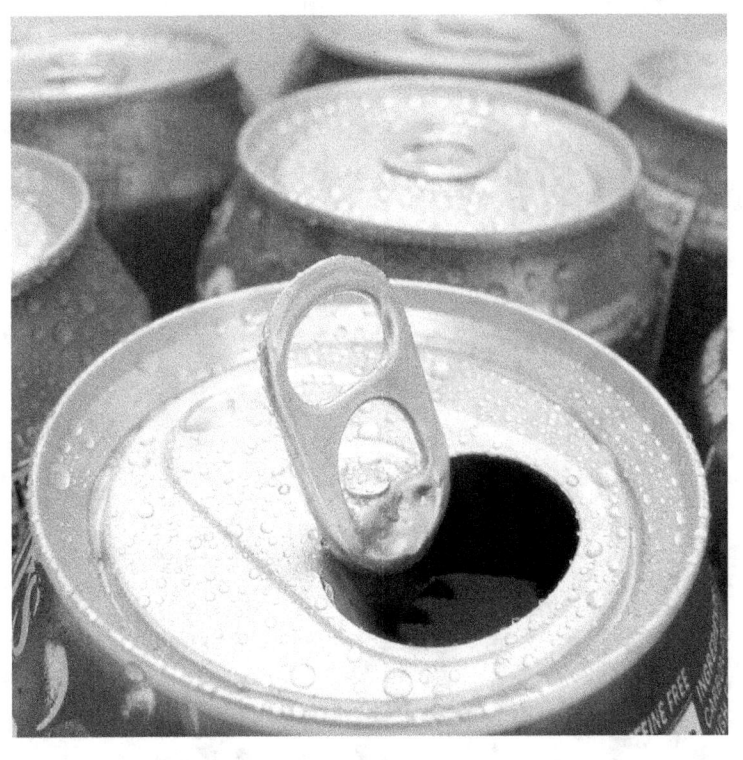

Try to cut soda out of your diet completely, even diet varieties contain artificial sweeteners and other additives that your body does not need

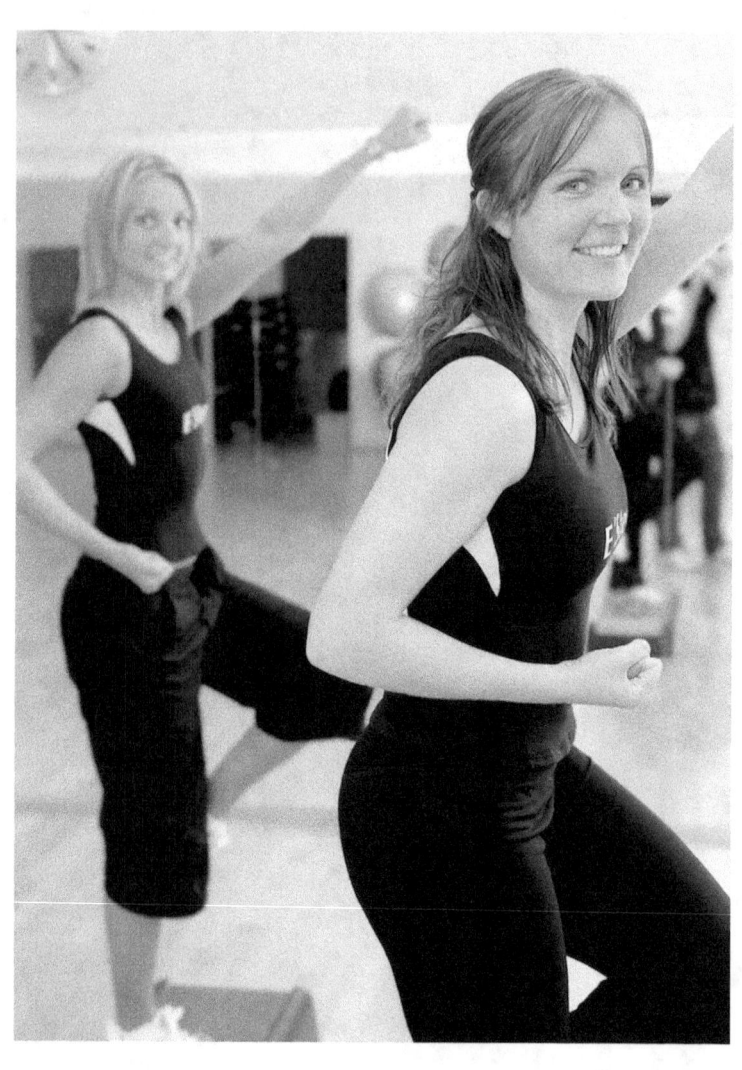

Join an exercise class if you feel more motivated
when working out with others

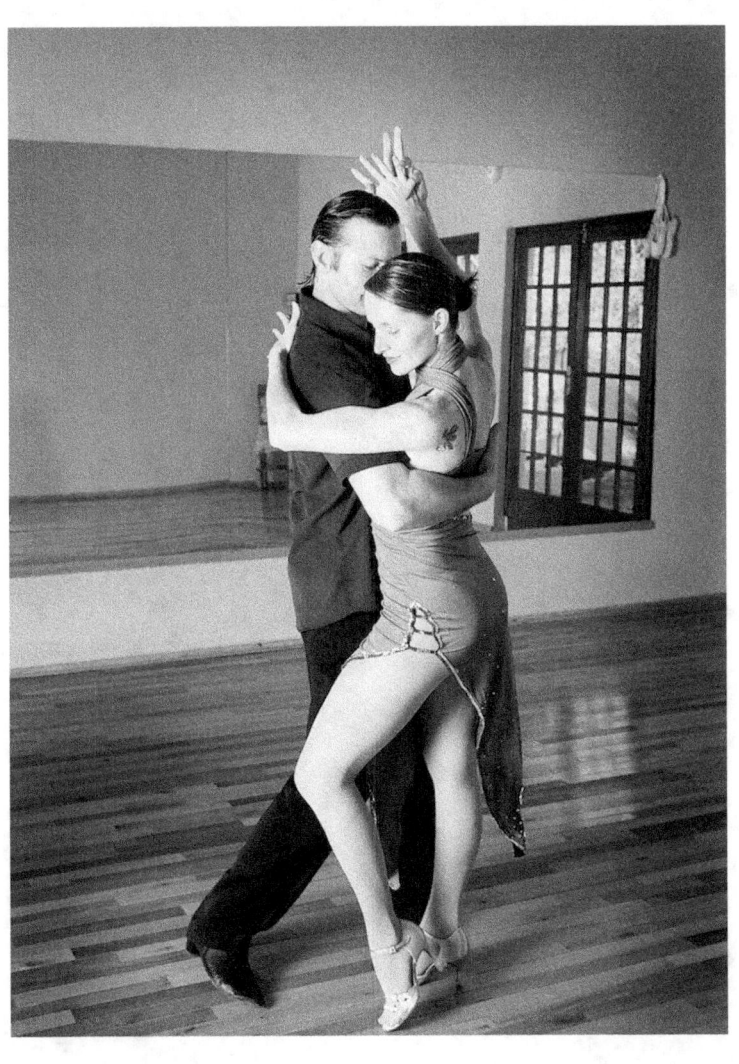

Join a dance class for an alternative way to incorporate
exercise into your life

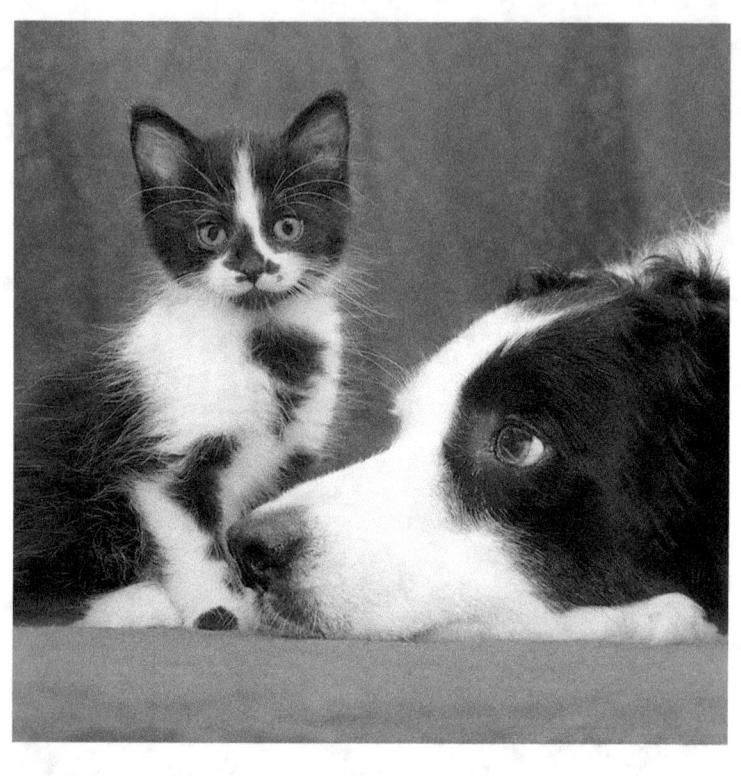

Owning and caring for animals can help reduce stress

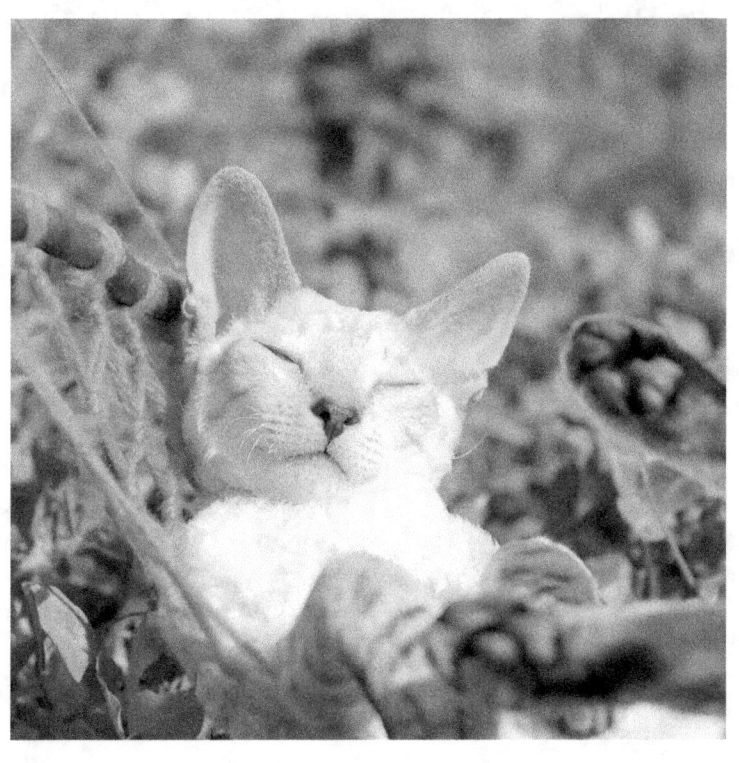

Reducing stress in your life will reduce your
susceptibility to colds and flu

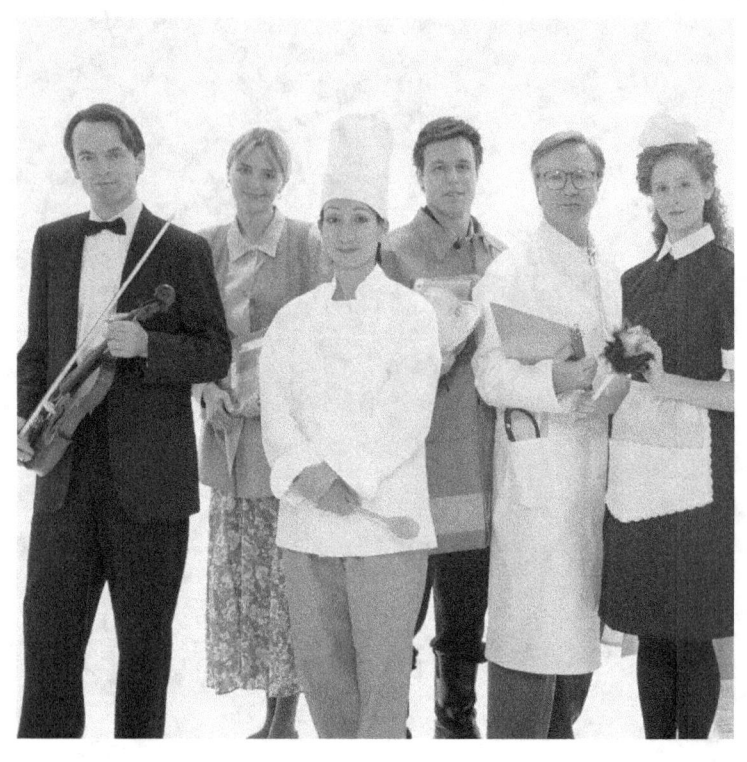

Learn who you are and have the courage to be that person

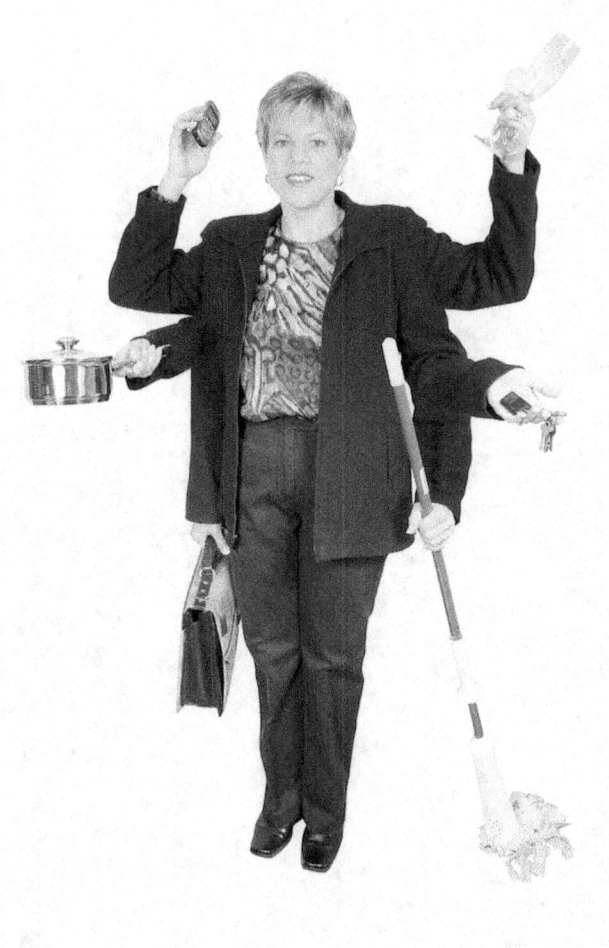

Personal expectations can be the cause of stress,
try to keep them realistic and achievable

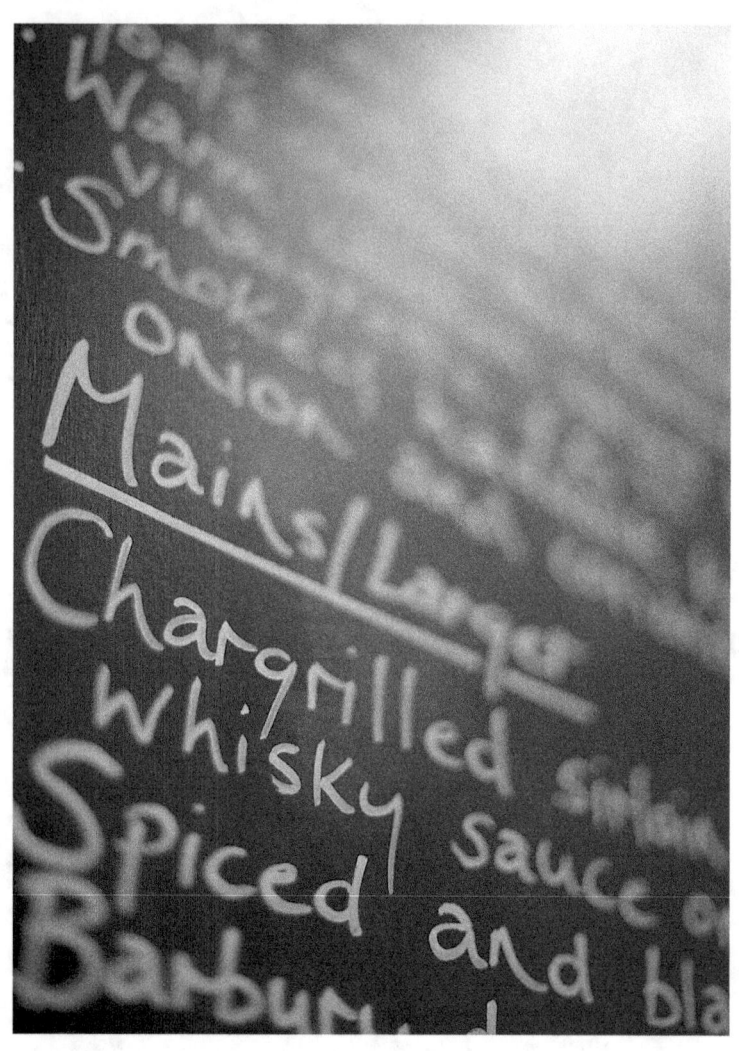

When eating out, try and check out the menu in advance to make a conscious decision to make a healthy choice

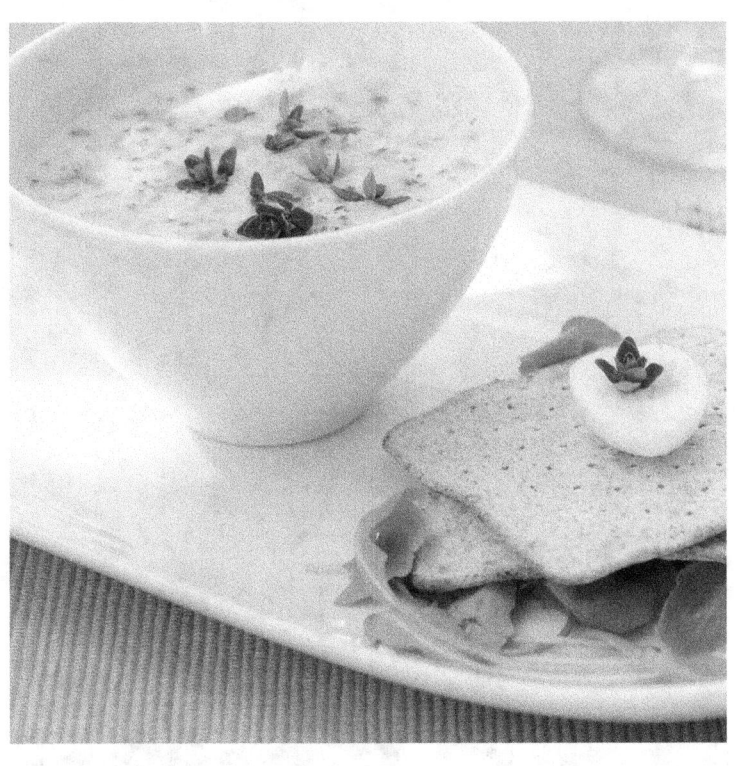

Try to eat several small portions of food a day rather than fewer large ones to increase metabolism and stabilize blood sugar levels

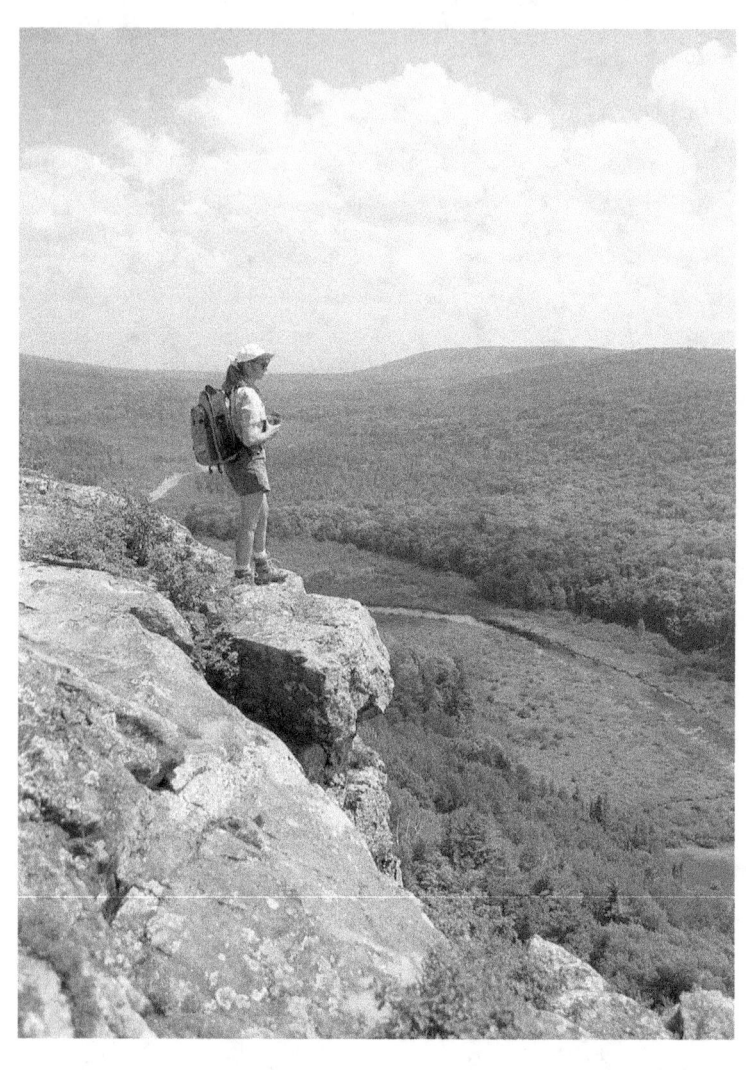

Buy a pedometer to encourage yourself to increase
your number of steps each day

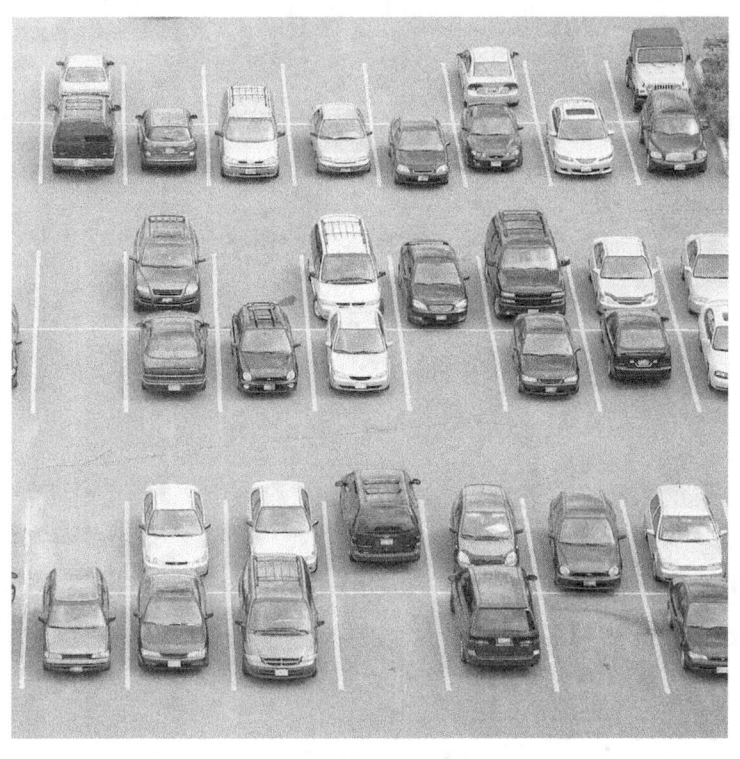

Park your car further away from work and stores
to get a little more exercise

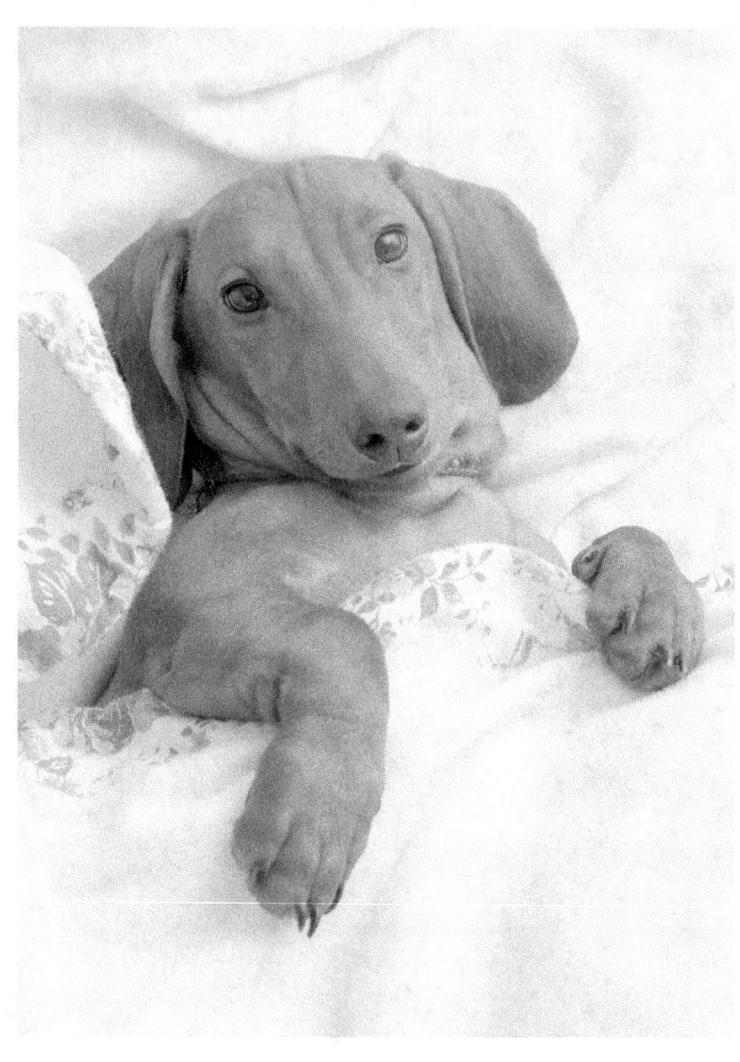

Try to go to bed and get up at the same time each day

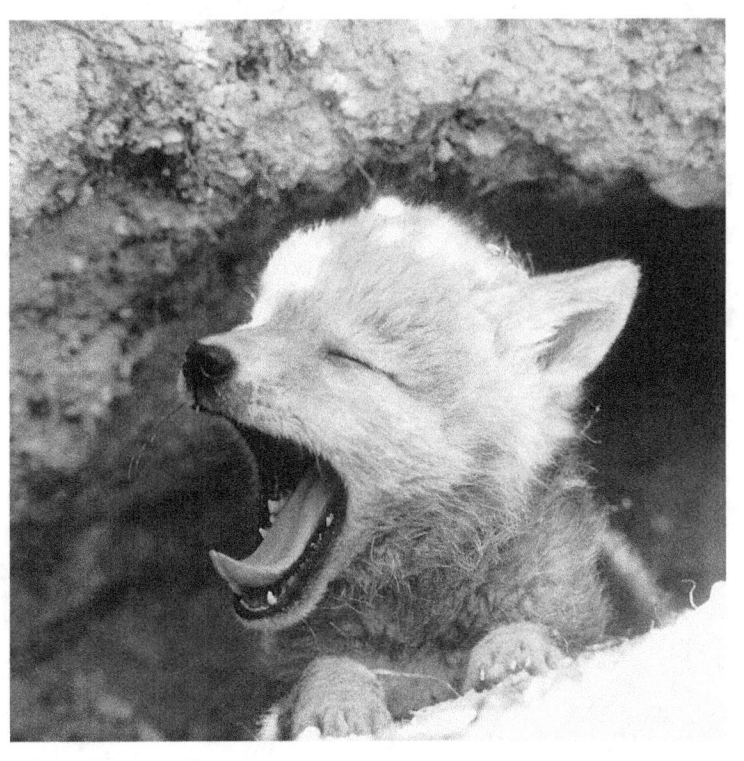

Get enough sleep, tired people eat more

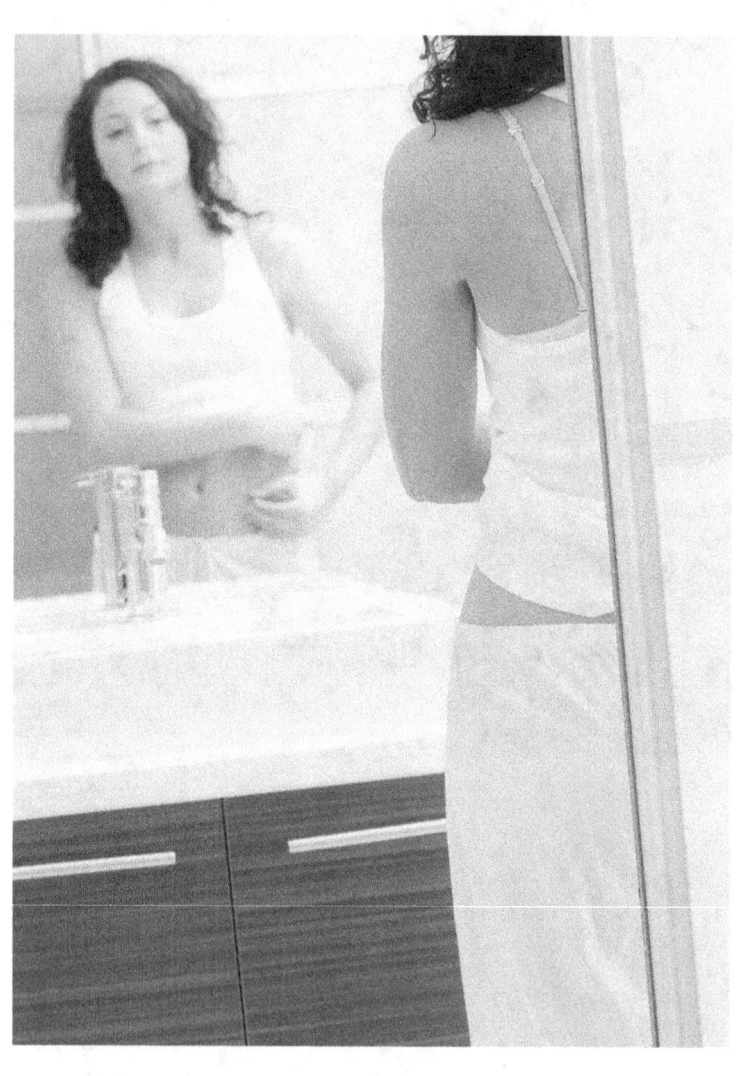

Stop picking on yourself

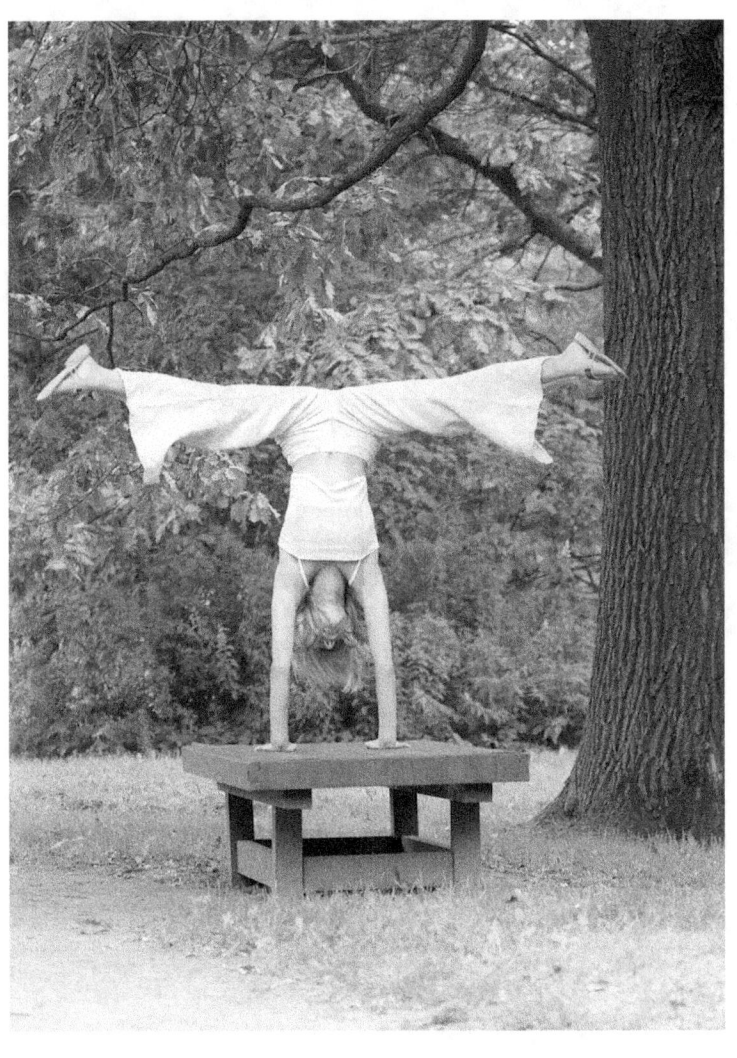

The body achieves what the mind believes

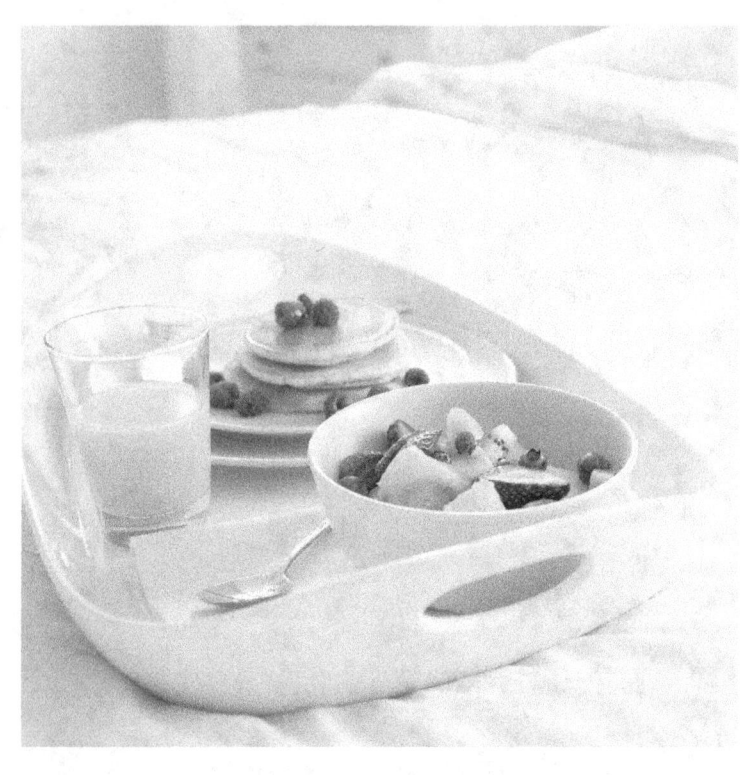

Never skip breakfast

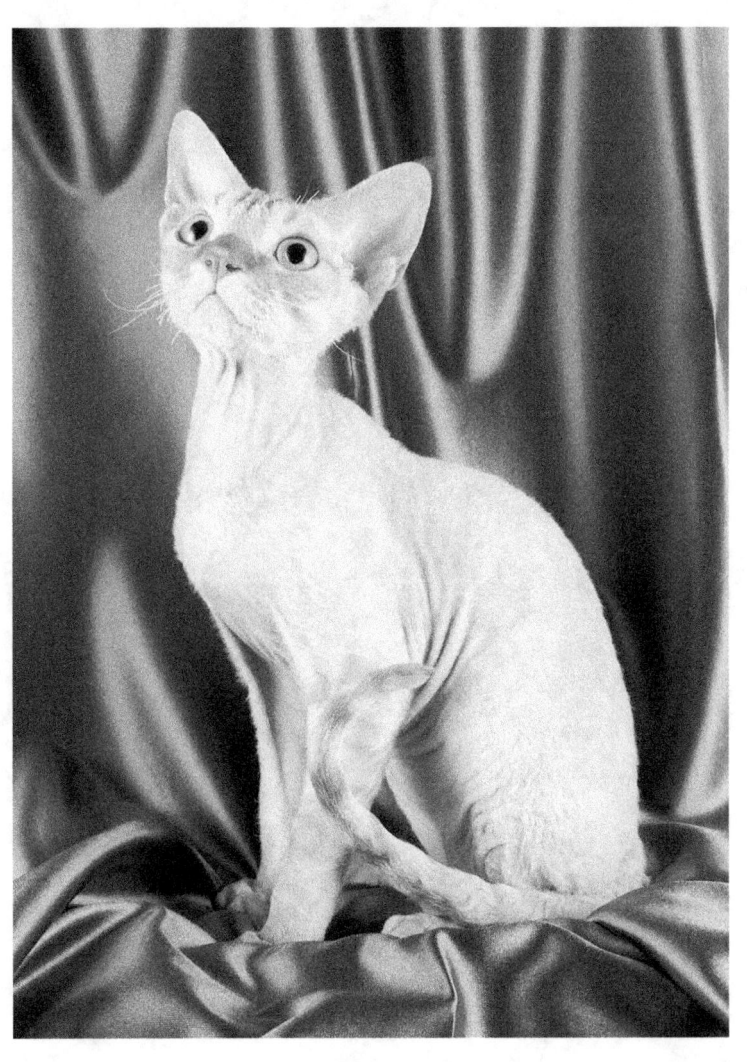

Don't starve yourself

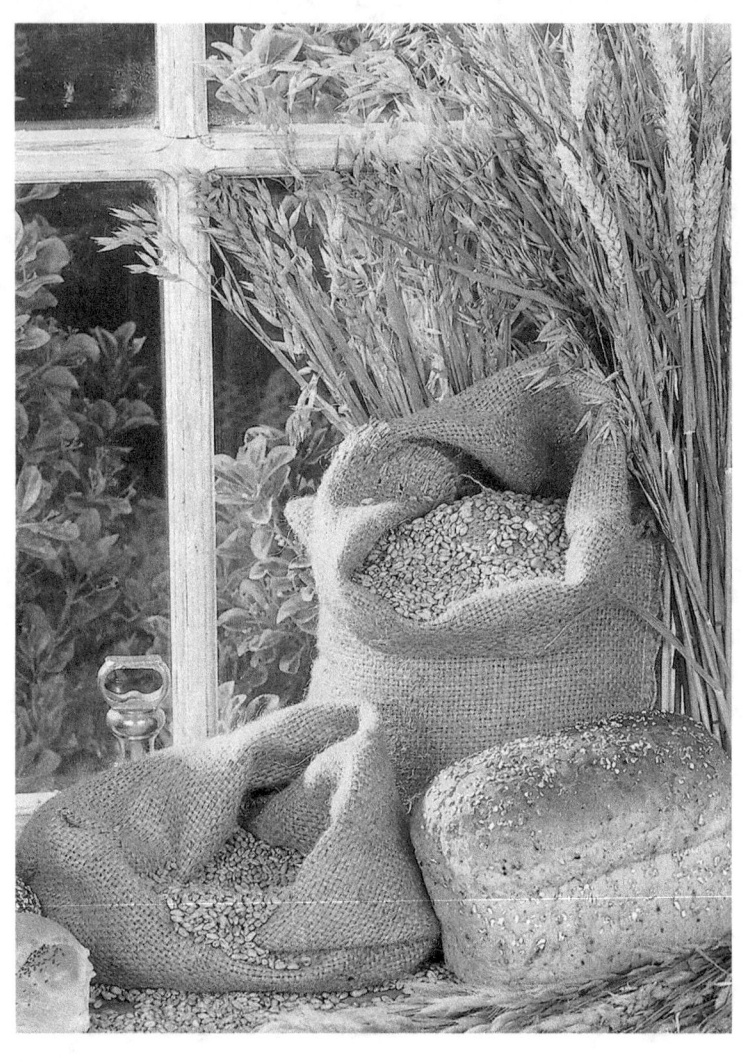

Replace refined bread and pasta products with whole wheat
to increase fiber in your diet

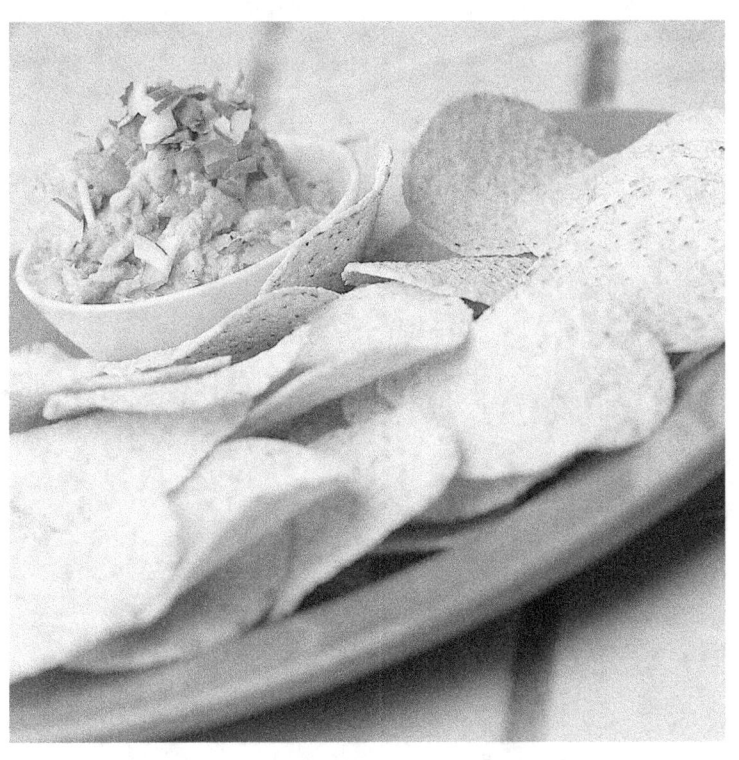

If you must eat chips choose baked varieties rather
than fried for less fat and calories

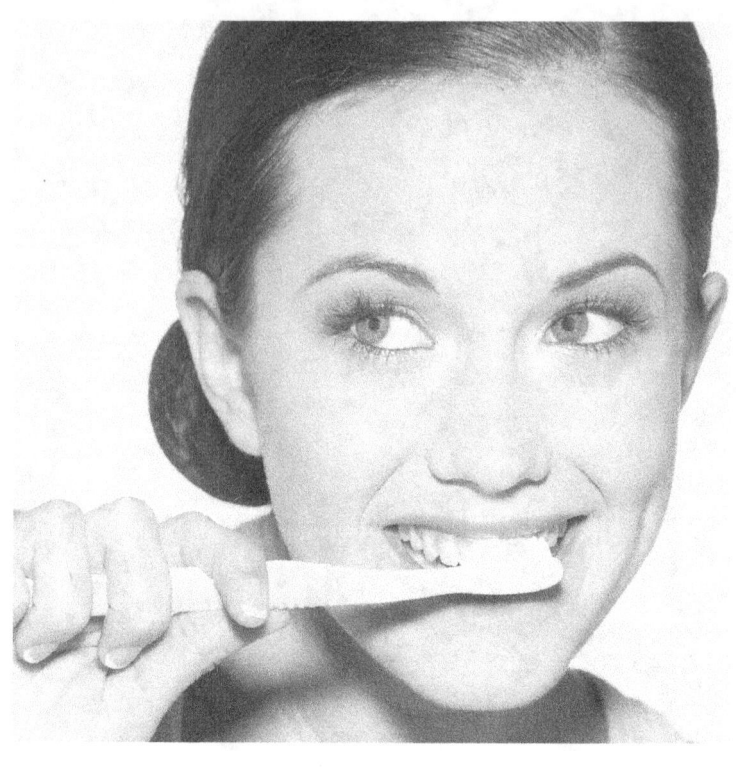

Brush your teeth in between meals to help prevent snacking

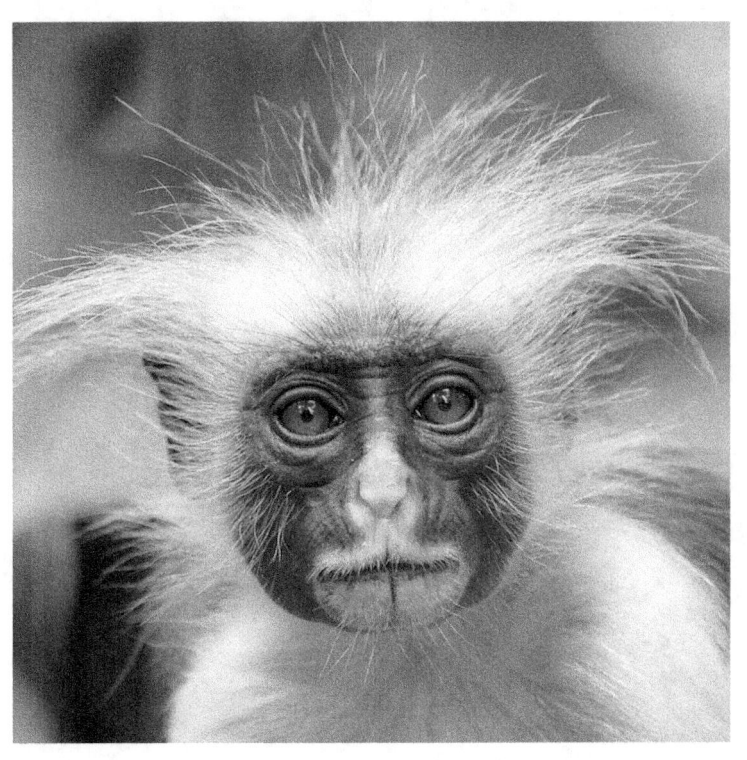

Switch toiletries to organic products to reduce
skin and hair drying chemicals

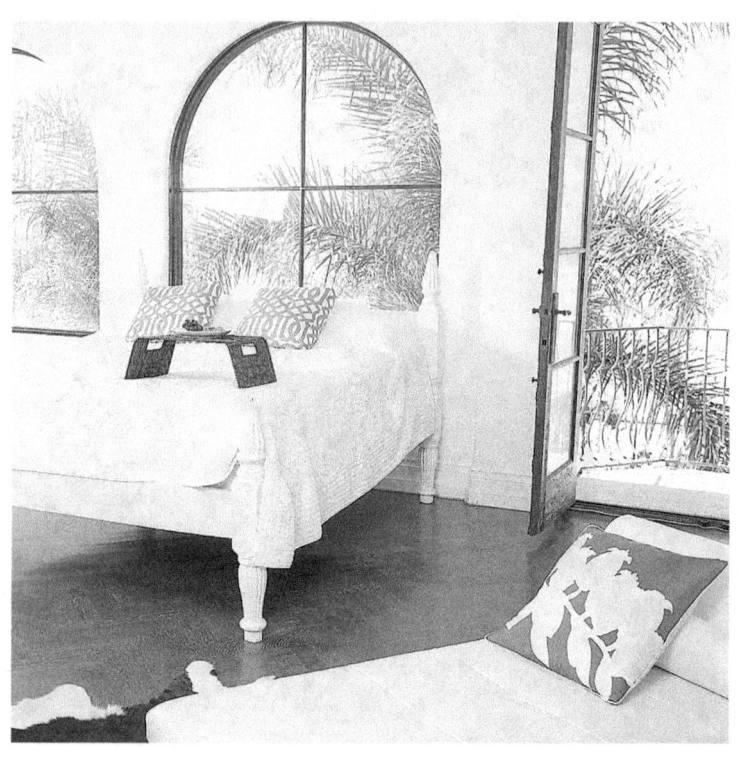

Open the windows in your home to let fresh air in

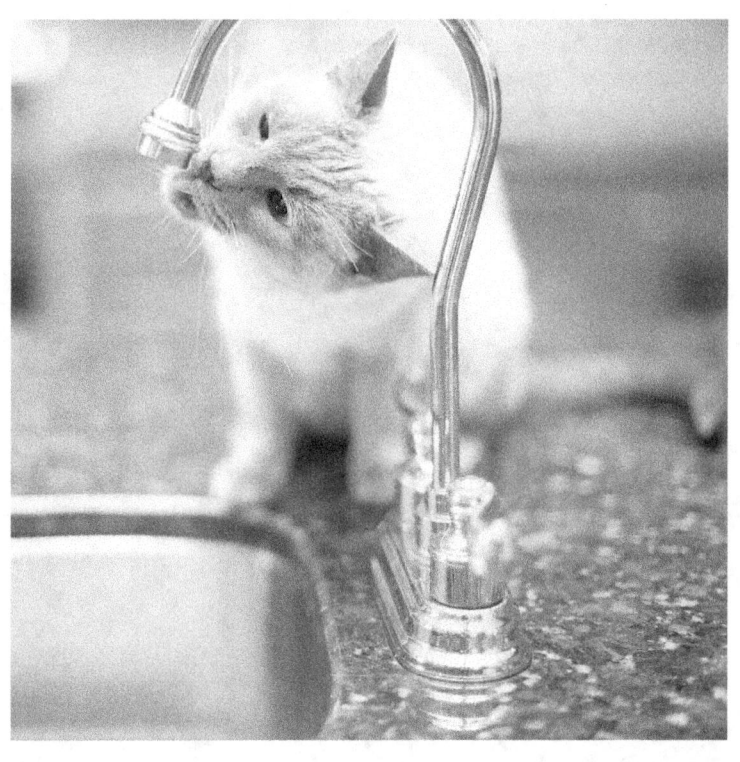

Try to keep pets off work surfaces where food is prepared

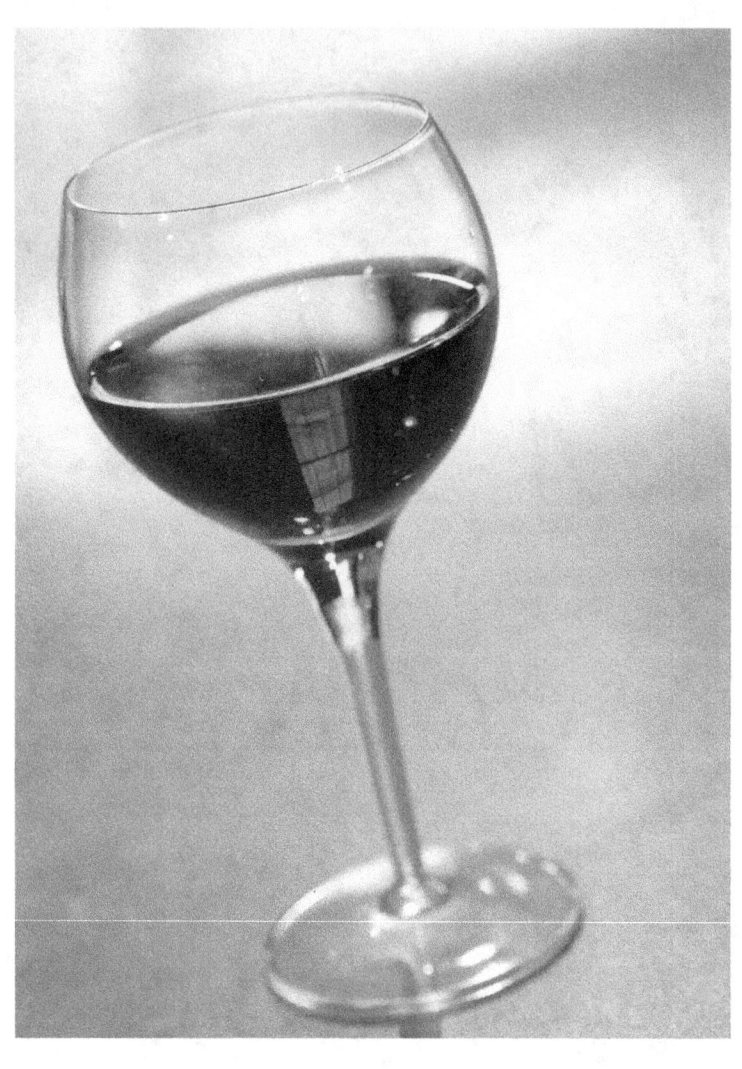

Limit calories through alcohol consumption. A glass of wine has fewer calories than a bottle of beer

Stop smoking

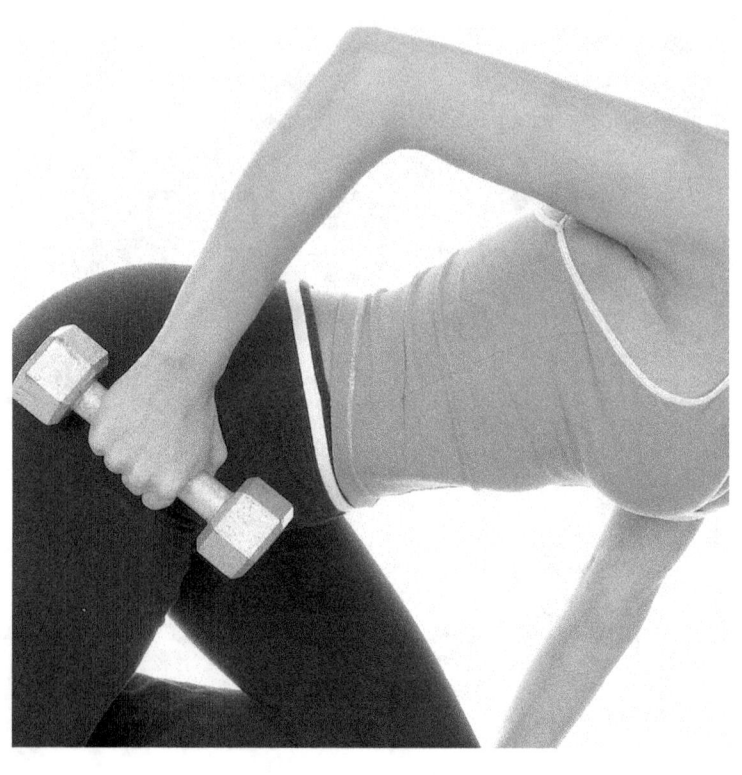

Don't be afraid of weight training, you will not grow
huge muscles over night, it takes a lot of effort to
build even a small amount of muscle

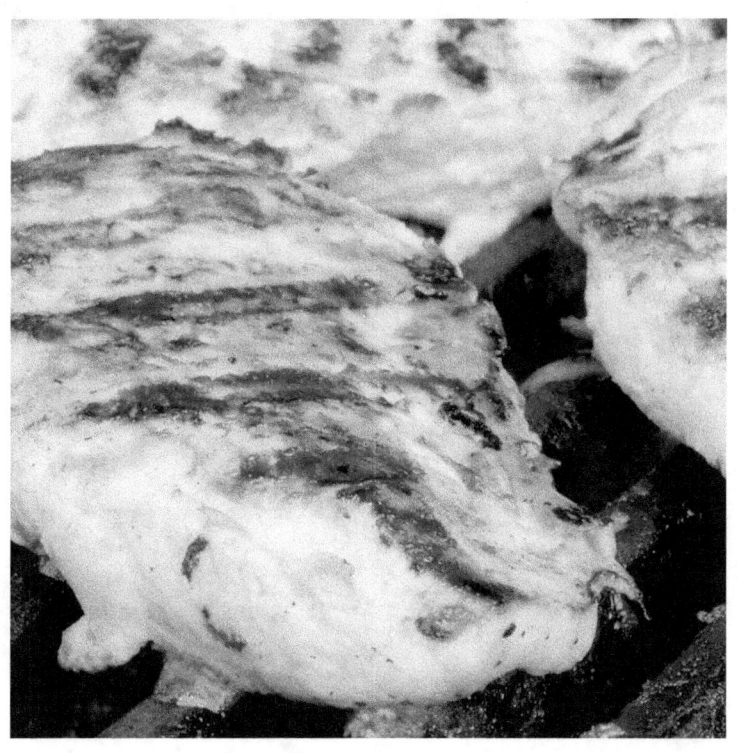

Try to consume a healthy source of protein within thirty
minutes of weight training to repair and build muscle

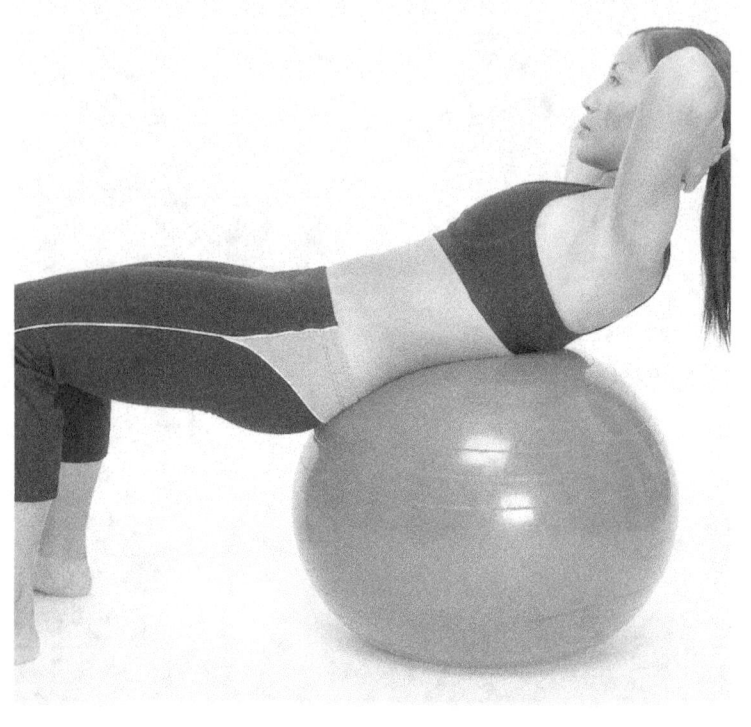

Subscribe to a fitness magazine to give you new exercise ideas

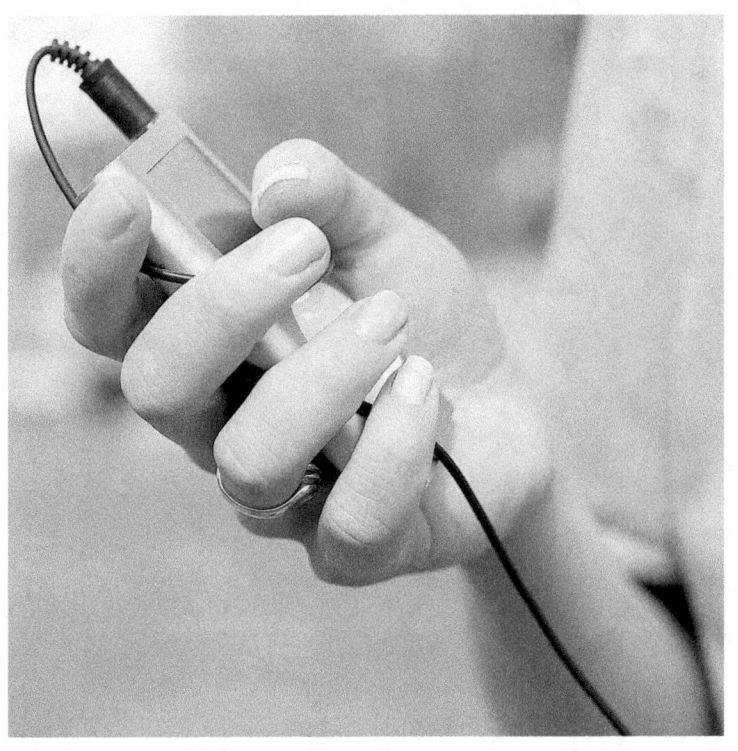

Using an MP3 player while you work out can keep you
motivated and make you exercise for longer

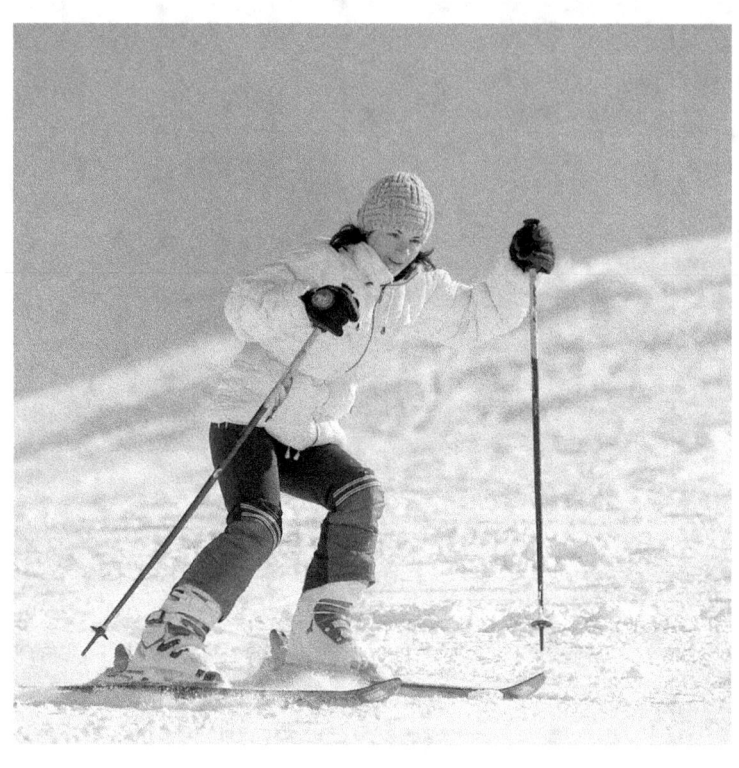

Busy people don't have time to overeat,
keep busy

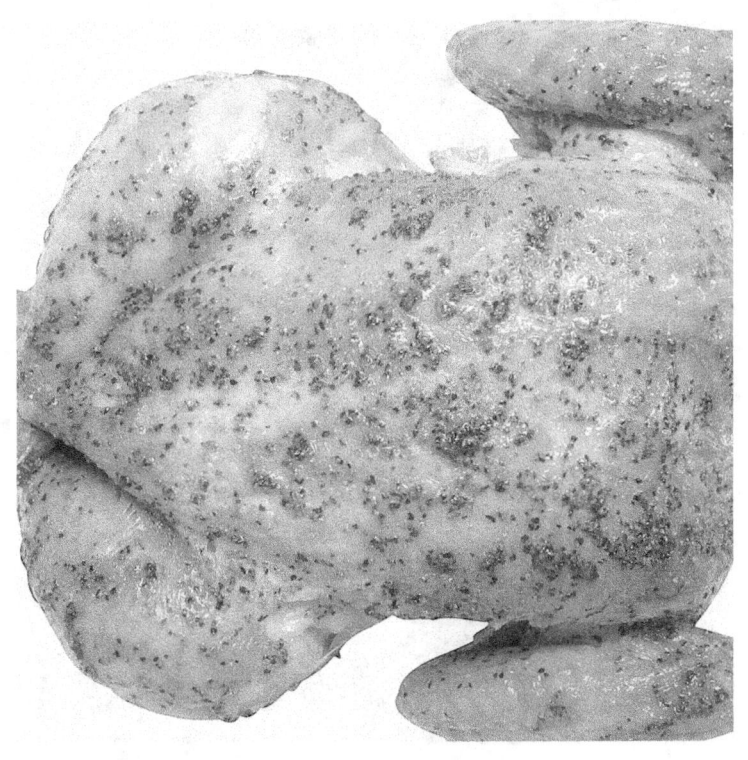

Buy a ready cooked chicken and pre-washed salad
if you want a healthy dinner in a rush

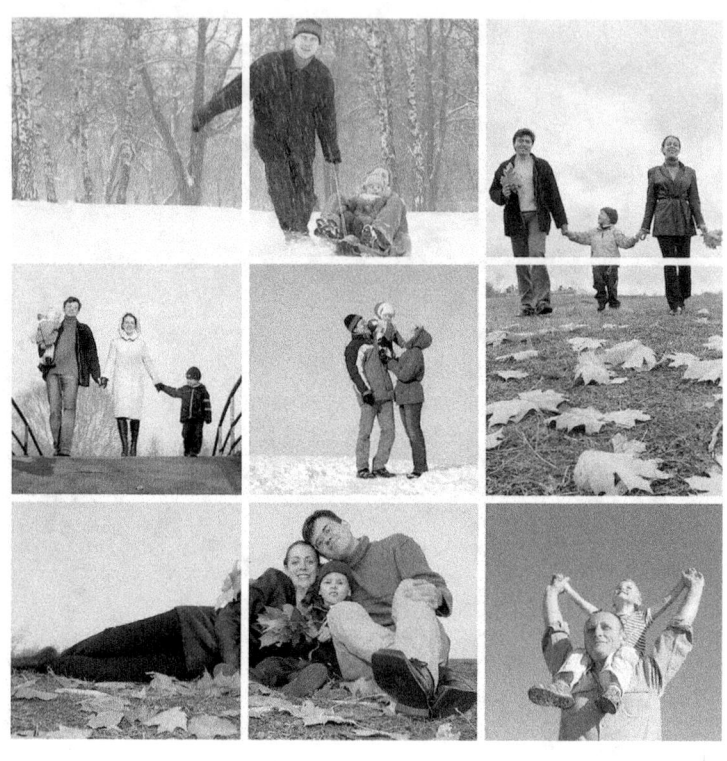

Set limits on work and family demands

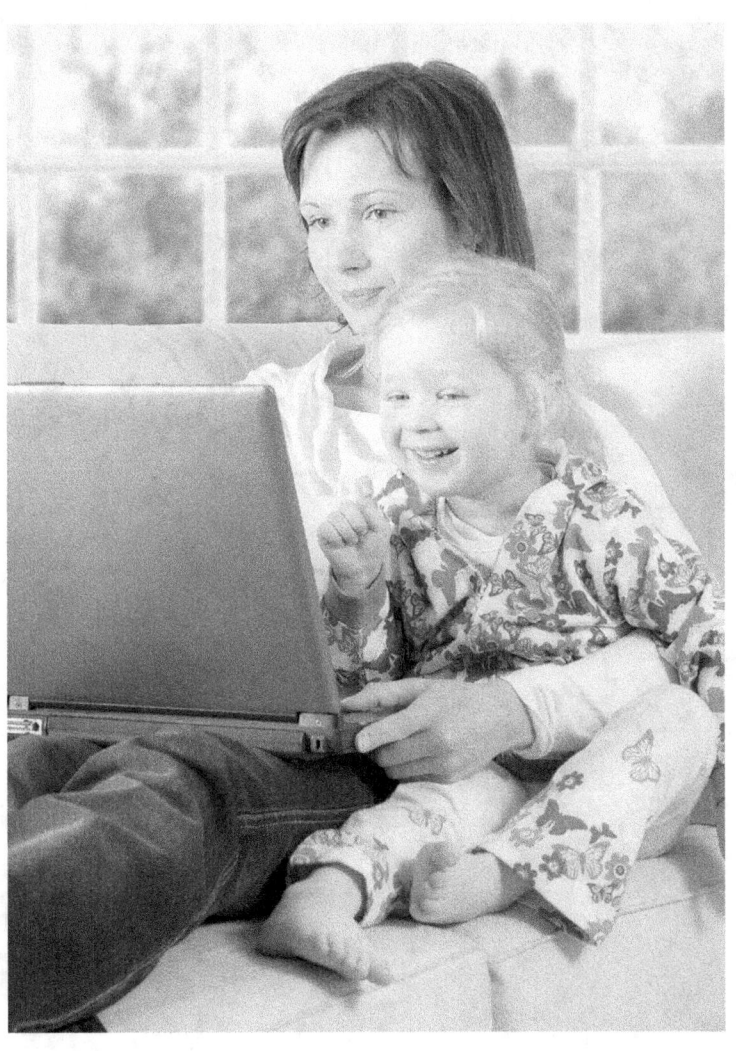

Try to maintain a healthy work-life balance

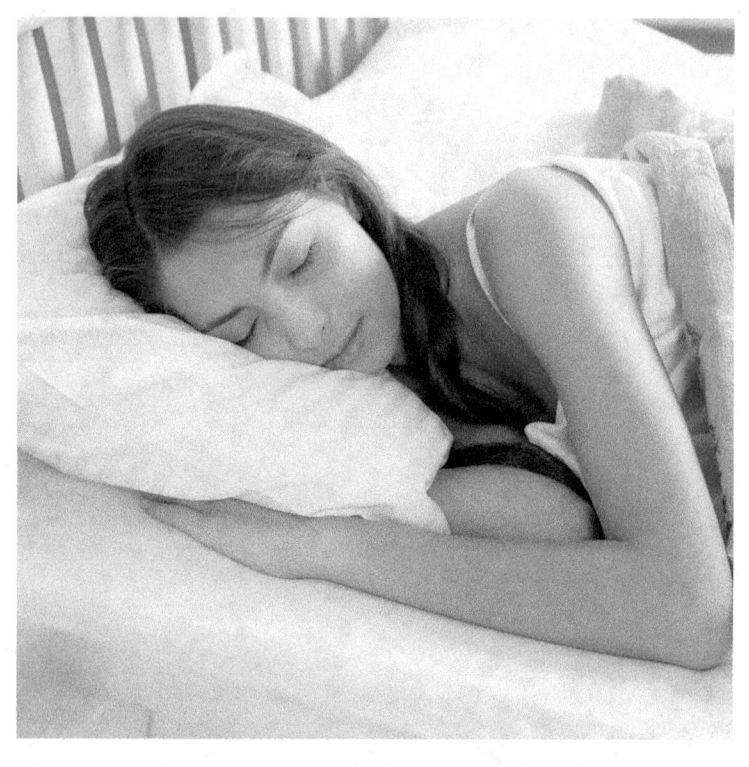

Don't eat anything within two hours of going to bed

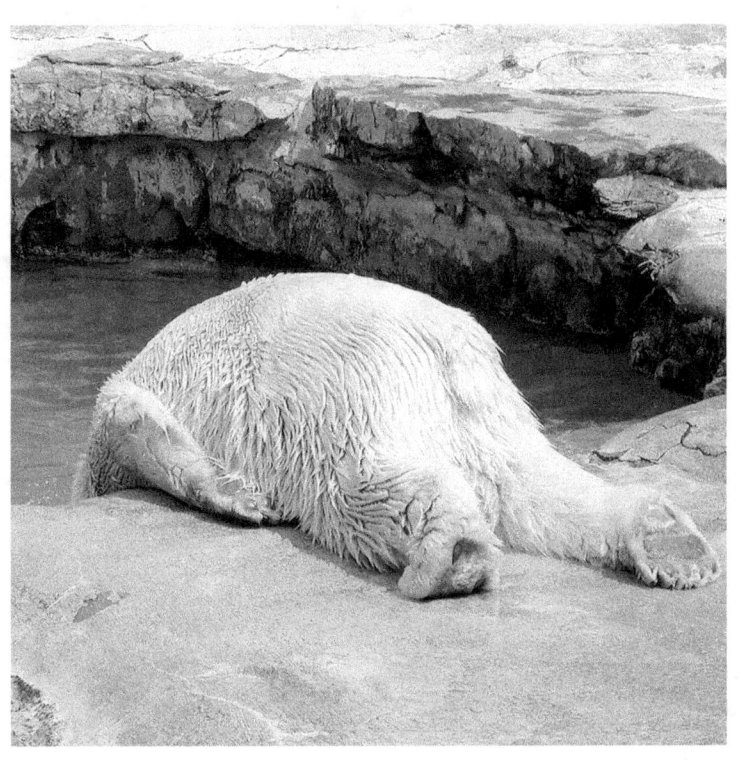

If you feel tired and unwell, rest.
Your body needs energy to recover

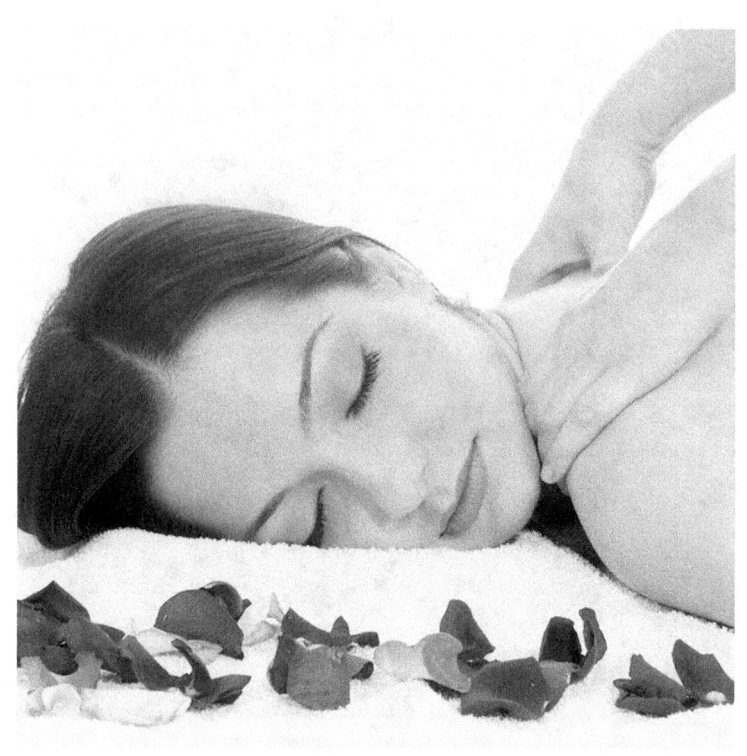

Get a massage to relieve your body of tension

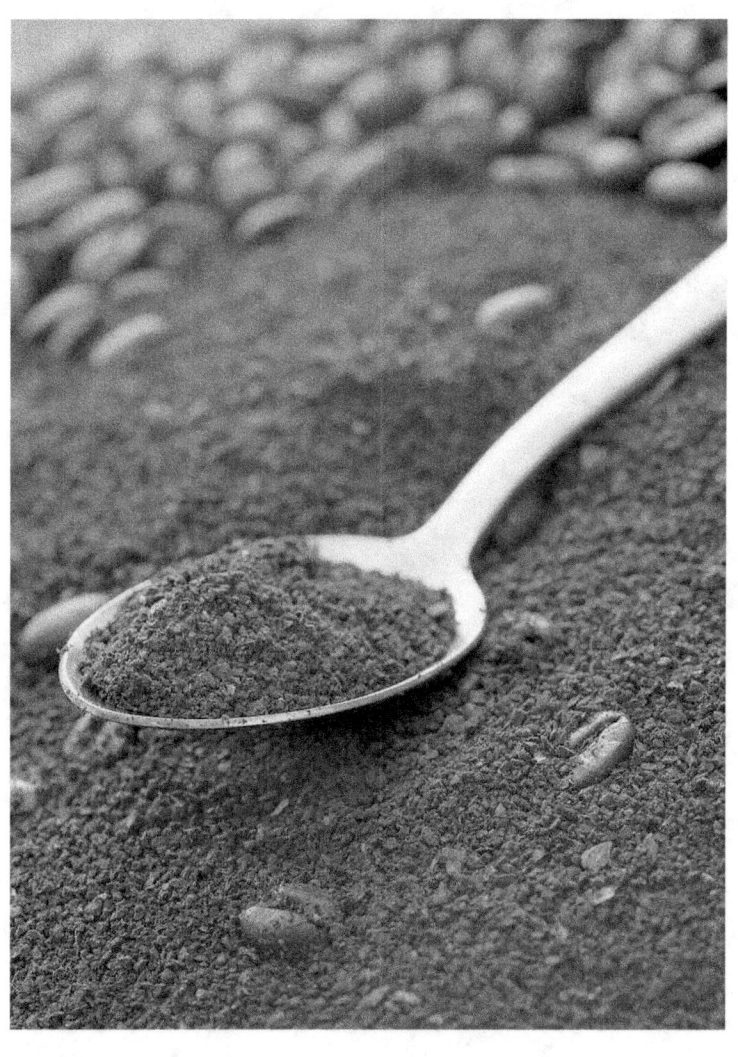

Reduce caffeine intake if you are prone to anxiety

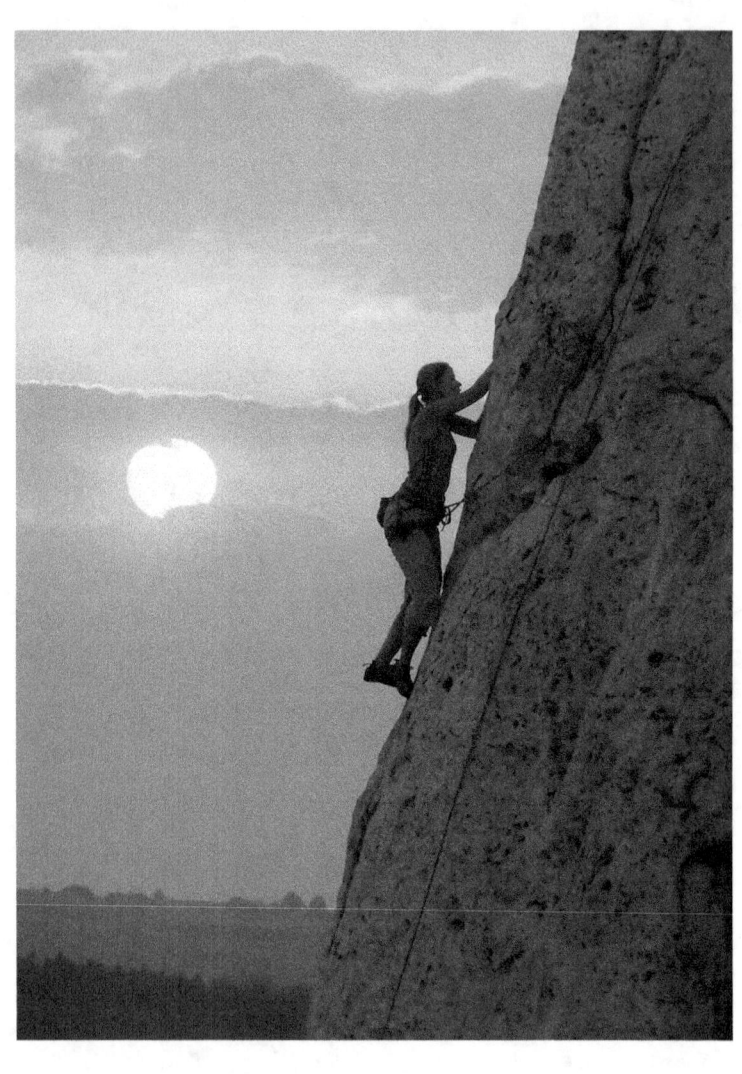

Allow commitment to fuel your determination

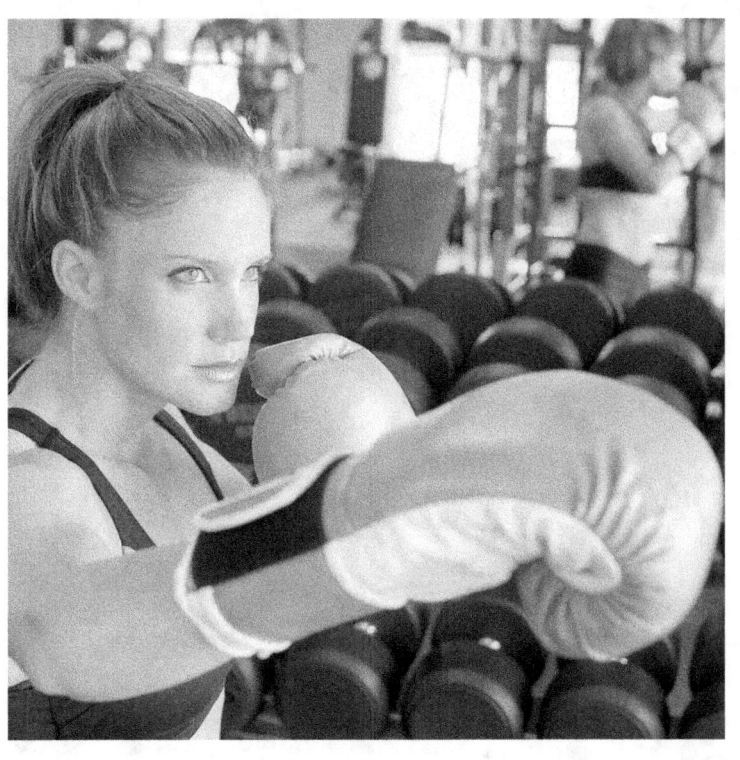

You do have the power to change

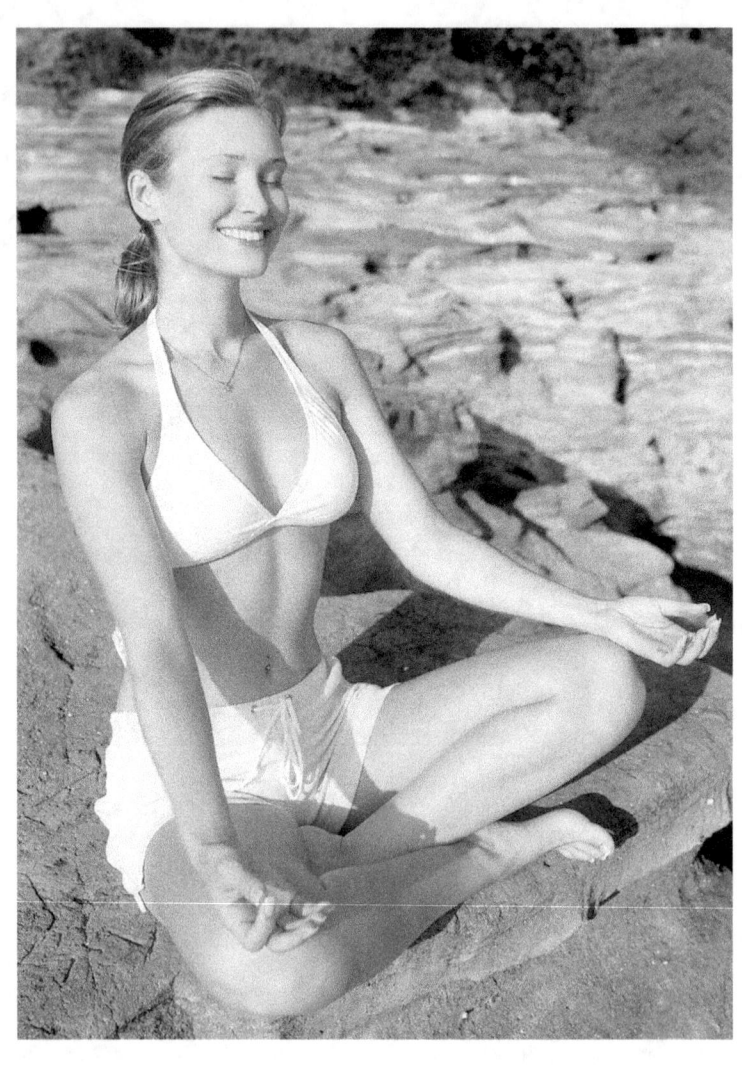

Your thoughts will be reflected in your body,
so think positively

www.ingramcontent.com/pod-product-compliance
Lightning Source LLC
Chambersburg PA
CBHW060423290526
45791CB00002B/850